BAILLIÈRE'S
SELF-ASSESSMENT FOR NURSES

Revise General Nursing
1

Other books by the same authors:

Revise General Nursing 2 covers the following topics:

- Care of the elderly patient
- Care of the patient with a sensory impairment
- Care of the female patient and her reproductive system
- Care of the patient with problems of the renal and urinary systems
- Care of the patient approaching death

Revise General Nursing 3 covers the following topics:

- Care of the patient with respiratory problems
- Care of the highly dependent patient
- Care of the patient with problems of body image
- Care of the sick child
- Care of the patient with problems of the nervous system

Baillière's Nursing Study Aids *Crosswords for Revision*—30 crosswords to help students learn, covering the following topics:

Abdominal surgery; anaemia; ante-natal care; anorexia nervosa; asthma; cardiac failure; cerebrovascular accident; cholecystitis; chronic bronchitis; Crohn's disease; community care; diabetes mellitus; eczema; fractured femur; head injury; leukaemia; mastectomy; meningitis; myocardial infarction; nephrotic syndrome; non-accidental injury; paediatric gastroenteritis; peptic ulcer; psoriasis; pyloric stenosis; renal failure; rheumatoid arthritis; thyroidectomy; tonsillectomy; vaginal hysterectomy.

BAILLIÈRE'S
SELF-ASSESSMENT FOR NURSES

Revise General Nursing 1

Christina Cheetham
SRN, RSCN, RCNT, Cert. Ed., RNT
Senior Tutor
Charles West School of Nursing
Great Ormond St, London

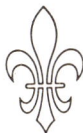

Joan Ramsay
SRN, DN(Lond.), Cert. Ed., RNT
Senior Tutor
Charles West School of Nursing
Great Ormond St, London

Baillière Tindall
London   Philadelphia   Toronto
Sydney   Tokyo   Hong Kong

Baillière Tindall	33 The Avenue
W. B. Saunders	Eastbourne, East Sussex BN21 3UN, England
	West Washington Square
	Philadelphia, PA 19105, USA
	1 Goldthorne Avenue
	Toronto, Ontario M8Z 5T9, Canada
	ABP Australia Ltd, 44–50 Waterloo Road
	North Ryde, NSW 2113, Australia
	Ichibancho Central Building, 22–1 Ichibancho
	Chiyoda-ku, Tokyo 102, Japan
	10/fl, Inter-Continental Plaza, 94 Granville Road
	Tsim Sha Tsui East, Kowloon, Hong Kong

First published 1987

Typeset by Photo·graphics
Printed and bound in Great Britain by Biddles Ltd,
Guildford, Surrey

British Library Cataloguing in Publication Data
Cheetham, Christina
    Revise general nursing 1.—
    (Baillière's self-assessment for nurses)
    1. Nursing—Problems, exercises, etc.
    I. Title II. Ramsay, Joan III. Series
    610.73'076   RT55

ISBN 0–7020–1192–4

Contents

Preface

The aim of this series of books is to provide the learner with an active means of independently evaluating his/her knowledge and understanding of patient care.

The books are intended for RGN students as a way of consolidating their previous knowledge. They could be used at the end of each unit of learning or as an aid to revision at the end of training.

It is probable that with the recent development of the state final examination, individual hospitals will have differing methods of assessment. However, whatever form of assessment is used, these books should provide a useful means for the learner to evaluate his/her own knowledge and understanding.

The three books are all sub-divided into five chapters, each concerned with a particular patient problem. The wide range of experience encountered by the learner during her training is covered within these chapters. Each chapter consists of a number of short case-histories and related questions.

The questions are concerned with the assessment, planning, implementation and evaluation of individual patients' care. The concepts of holistic nursing and research are seen as important aspects throughout. Suggested answers to questions are given after each case history.

Application of knowledge and problem-solving is seen as more important than recall of facts. This form of revision ensures that the learner understands the rationale for nursing care, and is able to be adaptable in different situations.

Acknowledgement must be made to the support and invaluable assistance given by Ms Richenda Milton-Thompson of Baillière Tindall.

Thanks also go to Mrs Susanne Walker and Mrs Maggie Wisby for typing the manuscript.

C. Cheetham

J. Ramsay

Introduction:
How to Use this Book

- This book has been designed to help you learn by yourself. You will find that it is divided into five chapters, each relating to a particular patient problem. Some you will have come across already; some you may meet later in your career. You might prefer to look at the problems you are familiar with first, as the sections do not interrelate, and can be taken in any order.
- The book is primarily intended as a consolidation of your previous theoretical and practical experiences. Therefore, you may wish to do some preparatory reading or revision before you tackle any of the case-histories. You may also use them as a pre-test of your knowledge. You may know more than you think!
- Questions are worded differently. To help you decide the most appropriate way to answer each you may like to spend some time familiarizing yourself with the commonly used words as shown below:

  Define: to state precisely your meaning of
  Describe: to give an account or representation of, in your own words
  Discuss: to investigate, examine by argument (i.e. by logical discussion), to sift or debate ideas and to reach your conclusion
  Explain: to make plain, interpret or account for; to give the reasons for your actions
  Identify: to determine the individual characteristics of
  List: to give an item-by-item record
  Outline: to provide a draft account, giving the main reasons or general principles of a subject
  State: to present in a brief, concise format

- The style of your answers is entirely up to you. You do not have to write a timed essay; notes will do. However, we do suggest some kind of written response as educational research shows that this significantly improves memory. Any help in remembering must be worth using!

- Do not worry if your answers are slightly different to those given. Our answers are not intended to be the only correct ones, but do contain the essential points. Also, we realize that each hospital has its own local practices. You may have to adapt our answer to meet your own hospital procedure.
- You will find that some topics are very specialized. If you have not had experience in these specialities you may prefer to use such case-histories to extend your knowledge rather than as a basis for revision.
- You will also find that some questions in some case-histories relate to ward management and teaching junior colleagues. You may wish to omit these questions until you have had experience in these areas.
- We hope that you find this way of studying useful, and, most importantly, enjoyable! If so, you may be interested in the companion volumes to this book.

1 Care of the Patient with Problems of the Heart and Circulation

1.1 Mr King—a middle-aged man who has had a myocardial infarction

Mr Reg King, aged 52 years, is a telecommunications engineer. He has been admitted to ward after a diagnosis of acute myocardial infarction has been made.

On admission Mr King is conscious but severely shocked. He is pale and sweating and complaining of nausea. Analgesia has been administered in the accident and emergency department.

1 What preparations should be made before Mr King's arrival on the ward?
2 How would you explain the significance of the observations made on Mr King during his first 24 hours in the ward?
3 What should you say to Mrs King when she comes to see her husband?
4 How would you explain the pathophysiology of a myocardial infarction to a junior colleague?
5 Describe the role of the nurse in the promotion of rest for Mr King during his first 48 hours in hospital.
6 Describe Mr King's gradual return to mobility.

Four days after admission, Mr King is sitting in a chair talking to his wife, when he suddenly collapses.

7 What features would indicate that Mr King had had a cardiac arrest?
8 As the nurse in charge of the ward, describe in order of priority how you would manage Mr King's arrest.

Mr King is successfully resuscitated and after a further period of rest is ready to get out of bed again and re-mobilize himself. However, he is very anxious about his heart function and fearful of another heart attack.

9   Explain the psychological problems of the coronary patient and how anxiety (such as that felt by Mr King) may be avoided.

10   Describe the advice Mr King will need before discharge.

1.1 Answers

1 The following should be made ready:
   - a firm-based bed in case of cardiac arrest
   - a bed within easy observation of the nurses' station
   - resuscitation equipment nearby but not within the patient's view; oxygen and suction in working order by the bedside
   - a cardiac monitor ready for use, facing away from the patient

2 The main purpose of closely observing the coronary patient is to detect changes in the patient's condition which may indicate complications of myocardial infarction, usually arrhythmias of an electrical nature. Undetected, these complications could cause death. Also cardiogenic shock, caused by decreased cardiac output and inadequate tissue perfusion, occurs in 10–15% of patients following a myocardial infarction.

   These complications can be monitored by:
   - $\frac{1}{2}$–**1-hourly blood pressure and pulse**. Further hypotension and tachycardia indicates worsening cardiac function. The pulse must also be observed as rate and rhythm irregularities may indicate a failing or erratic heart action.
   - **Colour and respirations**. Pallor or cyanosis and dyspnoea are indications of a failing heart; oxygen is no longer being circulated sufficiently.
   - **4-hourly temperature**. Fever is rare initially after an infarction. However, a moderate pyrexia (not exceeding 38°C) usually occurs after the first 24 hours as a reaction to tissue damage. A high temperature may be indicative of complications such as pericarditis.
   - **Fluid intake and output**. Acute renal failure can be a complication of myocardial infarction as a result of prolonged hypotension and consequent renal ischaemia. A careful watch for anuria or oliguria must be kept.
   - **General condition**. Cold or clammy skin is indicative of a poor peripheral circulation. The patient should be observed for non-verbal indications of pain such as rigidity, pallor and facial grimaces.

3 Mrs King should be taken to a quiet, private place before she sees her husband. It should be explained to her that her husband has had a heart attack. It should also be explained that he is fairly stable, but that she may be

shocked to see him looking so ill. (If a cardiac monitor is being used she must be warned about this—a routine way of monitoring his heart action.)

Mrs King will also need to know that the first 48 hours are crucial in Mr King's management. He must be allowed complete physical and psychological rest. For this reason it is best if she is the only person to visit at this time. She can come at any time but should try not to tire him or worry him about anything.

Mrs King should be assured that she will be kept up-to-date with Mr King's progress, and she should be escorted to the bedside.

Following her visit, the nurse should talk to her again to see if she has any further questions and to allow her to express her feelings. The necessary information should be obtained to complete her husband's nursing assessment. In doing this, problems such as caring for small children while she is visiting or taking time off work may be revealed. Help may then be able to be offered.

4   First check your colleague's present knowledge. Ask her if she can draw a diagram of the heart showing the coronary circulation (see Fig. 1). Ensure that she is aware that the heart muscle is termed the myocardium. Then you can explain that a myocardial infarction is caused by a plaque of atherosclerosis which narrows or obstructs the coronary arteries. This obstruction prevents blood and oxygen from flowing to the myocardium. If a large portion of the myocardium has been affected, the heart will be unable to function at all and the patient will die immediately. In other patients the portion of myocardium affected will be relatively small and the remaining myocardium will continue to contract. Cardiac function, although disturbed, can also continue.

An acute myocardial infarction upsets the heart's pumping mechanism. Loss of function of part of the myocardium decreases stroke volume and cardiac output. Often, conduction of electrical impulses is also impaired.

5   The aims in the care of the patient who has had a myocardial infarction include reducing cardiac workload to allow healing and prevent extension of the infarction or complications.

The nurse can help to promote rest in several ways:

- **Bedrest** It should be explained to the patient that rest will help to heal his damaged heart and develop the surrounding circulation. He should stay in bed and not have to reach for anything. His locker and personal

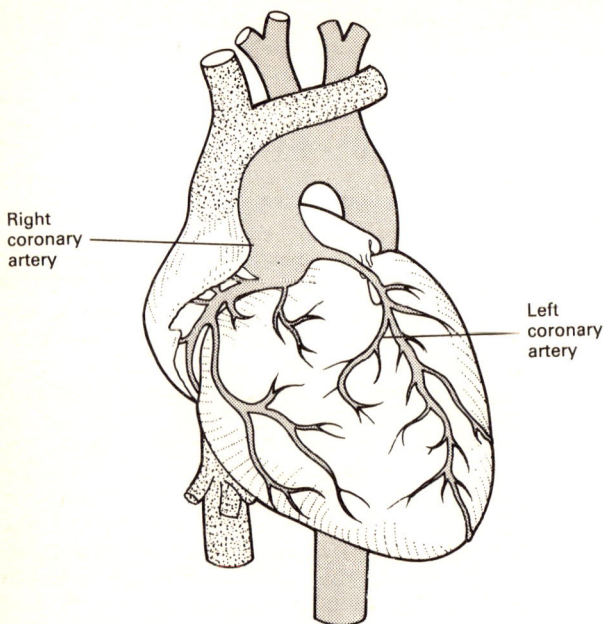

Fig. 1   External view of the heart illustrating the coronary circulation.

belongings should be within easy reach, together with the call-bell. He should be assured that he can call the nurse at any time if he needs anything.

Nursing care should be organized so that the patient is disturbed as little as possible. Any care (e.g. bed bathing) that may tire the patient should be done slowly with allowance for rest periods during care.

Visitors should be restricted to the next-of-kin, who should be warned not to overtire the patient.

- **Reduction of anxiety** Mental rest is as important as physical rest. The patient should be reassured about his condition and all care and treatment should be explained to him.

A calm, competent approach will help to reassure the patient. The nurse should give him an opportunity to express any fears or anxieties.

If the patient is very anxious and unable to relax, sed-

ation such as diazepam 2–5 mg 8-hourly may be prescribed.

- **Environment** Ideally, the patient should be in a situation
within the ward where he can rest easily, away from
noise and bustle and from other acutely ill patients who
may cause him anxiety.
- **Physical rest** Other means of reducing cardiac workload
are:

  1 providing an easily digestible diet

  2 maintaining the patient's normal bowel habit to prevent straining at stool. Use of the commode involves less
  energy expenditure than getting on and off the bedpan.

6 Mr King will be able to remobilize gradually 48 hours after
admission, providing his temperature has returned to normal and he has had no further chest pain since his initial
attack.

   On his first day out of bed Mr King will be allowed to sit
in a chair for half-an-hour only in the morning and afternoon. On the second day he can sit out twice for an hour
each time and on the third day for 2 hours a time. On the
fourth day he will be able to sit out as much as he likes and
walk to the toilet. He can do as much as he likes on the
fifth day. On the sixth day he will be ready for discharge
providing he has remained apyrexial and free of chest pain.

7 • Sudden loss of consciousness
  • Extreme pallor/cyanosis/greyness of skin
  • Absence of a major pulse (carotid or femoral)
  • Cessation of respirations
  • Dilated pupils

8 1 Call for help from the rest of your staff. When they reach
   you, delegate your most senior colleague to take Mrs King
   to the office and stay with her.

   Send a nurse to phone for the resuscitation team and
   to collect the resuscitation equipment on return from the
   telephone.

  2 Lower Mr King onto the floor.

  3 Clear his airway of any debris or obstruction (e.g. loose
   false teeth) and extend his jaw, while a colleague draws
   the curtains.

  4 Place your mouth over his (or over a guedel airway if
   available) to perform mouth-to-mouth resuscitation.
   Watch to ensure that his chest rises in response to your
   artificial respiration. Deliver several full breaths in quick
   succession initially.

  5 A colleague can then perform cardiac massage. You should

ensure that she places the heels of her hands, one on top of another, at right angles on the lower sternum. Downward compressions should depress the sternum by 1½–2 ". A rate of 60 compressions per minute should be maintained. After every five compressions she should pause to allow you to deliver one respiration.

6 Between respirations, evaluate the effectiveness of the cardiac massage by feeling the carotid pulse and observing for constriction of the pupils.

7 When the nurse returns with the resuscitation equipment, ask her to move the bed, chair and locker out of the way. It may be appropriate for her to move nearby patients and relatives away from the scene. She should then go round the ward and ensure that all the other patients are all right.

8 When the resuscitation team arrives and takes over artificial respiration, your second nurse can help the anaesthetist while you attach electrodes to monitor Mr King's heartbeat, prepare an infusion and draw up drugs as needed. Ensure that you keep a note of the drugs used.

9 When the resuscitation is over, ask the doctor to speak to Mrs King.

Arrange for restocking of the resuscitation trolley and record the arrest in Mr King's nursing records.

Inform your nurse manager of either the death of the patient or that you now have a critically ill patient. (You may require help for the evening shift or the transfer of the patient to the intensive care unit.)

Check that your staff are all right. Often junior staff can feel shaky and tearful after an arrest. They may need to talk about the situation and need reassurance that they coped well.

Then reassure the other patients about the occurrence.

9 **Psychological problems**

- **Denial of the illness** Denial relieves anxiety about dying, loss of good health and being a burden. Denial may result in the patient ignoring advice and refusing to rest or follow instructions.
- **Depression** The patient begins to feel sad and perhaps guilty about his illness because he is overweight or is a smoker.
- **Feelings of inadequacy** Men particularly may find the period of bed rest and dependency very threatening to their self-image and masculine role. This may be revealed by aggressive sexual behaviour.

- **Cardiac neurosis** This term is used to describe the anxiety of some coronary patients. Their anxiety becomes so overwhelming that they are afraid to do any kind of activity for fear of precipitating another attack.
  This can be avoided by:
  1 remaining calm and reassuring towards the patient to avoid communicating your fear
  2 giving the patient opportunities to voice his feelings and fears
  3 being very specific about how much activity the patient can do once he begins to get out of bed
  4 being positive about the future. Stress the number of patients who return to normal lives.

10 On discharge Mr King should take the following advice:
- Eat three small meals a day and eat them slowly. Avoid eating a lot of salty or fatty foods. Rushed, heavy meals put an extra strain on the heart. If overweight, he should reduce weight.
- Avoid situations or people which make him tense, upset or angry. In such moods the heart works faster.
- Plan his lifestyle to allow rest periods for his heart. He should try not to allow himself to be rushed. Sleep should be for 6–8 hours a night.
- Gradually increase his level of activity. Immediately after discharge he should get up and dress and walk as much as he did in hospital on level ground. Stairs should only be attempted once a day at this stage. This should be increased daily so that by the time he returns to clinic in 6 weeks he is achieving his usual level of activity.
- Avoid straining the heart by straining at stool, heavy lifting (anything heavier than a full kettle) or pushing and pulling heavy objects until seen in clinic.
- Not drive, return to work, play golf or any sport, or take an aeroplane trip until seen in clinic.
- Not smoke or drink in excess. Both habits will increase the chance of a further heart attack.
- Not have sex (in the first 6 weeks after the attack) if he is tired, angry or has just eaten or been drinking alcohol. In these events his heart is already overworking and may not be able to manage extra work. He should remember that it is normal for his heart to beat faster and for his breathing to speed up after sexual activity. This should return to normal shortly afterwards.
- Notify his general practitioner if he has any chest pain

or cramp-like pains in the jaw, neck, shoulder or arm, breathlessness, swelling of ankles or palpitations.

It is best to give Mr King these instructions in written form following your explanation so that he can refer to them at home.

1.2   Mr Westwood—an adult with hypertension

Mr Gerald Westwood, aged 45 years, is a police sergeant. He has been admitted to the ward for investigations of hypertension that was discovered during a routine medical examination. On admission he has a blood pressure of 180/110 mmHg.

Four-hourly recordings of Mr Westwood's blood pressure have been ordered, together with a 24-hour urine collection for creatinine. He is to be nursed at rest except for toilet purposes.

1   Describe how the assessment of Mr Westwood on admission may help in his investigations.
2   How would you explain hypertension to a junior colleague?
3   Describe the role of the nurse in ensuring the accuracy of Mr Westwood's blood pressure recordings.
4   Describe how you can ensure accuracy when given responsibility for Mr Westwood's 24-hour urine collection which is to commence at 10 a.m., Monday.

Mr Westwood's diagnosis is confirmed as essential hypertension. He has been prescribed propranolol 40 mg 8-hourly.

5   How would you explain Mr Westwood's diagnosis to him?
6   How would you describe to a junior colleague how propranolol acts and its possible side-effects?
7   How can the nurse evaluate the effects of Mr Westwood's drug therapy?
8   What nursing interventions may also help to reduce Mr Westwood's blood pressure?
9   What advice will be given to Mr Westwood on his discharge?
10   Discuss the prevention of hypertension for the general public.

1.2   Answers

1   Hypertension is divided into two main categories—primary (essential) and secondary hypertension.

   The cause of primary hypertension is unknown but many patients seem to have a predisposition to raised blood pressure because of their personality and/or lifestyle.

   During the admission interview the nurse may be able to elicit the following predisposing factors:
   - Is Mr Westwood a smoker?
   - Is Mr Westwood overweight?
   - Does he seem to manage stress well?
   - Does he have much time for rest and relaxation and sleep?

   Secondary hypertension indicates that the blood pressure is raised secondary to some other condition. The nurse may find the following information useful in identifying such a condition in the initial assessment of Mr Westwood:
   - **Urinalysis** Glycosuria may indicate mature-onset diabetes mellitus. Proteinuria and/or haematuria may indicate renal disease.
   - **Nursing history** If the patient reveals problems such as polyuria and thirst, he may have diabetes or aldosteronism. Headaches and palpitations may indicate an adrenal tumour. Attacks of loin pain and pain on passing urine may be symptomatic of pyonephritis.
   - **Observation** The presence of oedema may be the result of renal disease or Cushing's syndrome.

2   First check your junior colleague's present knowledge. Ensure that she understands what is meant by blood pressure. Also ensure that she can define hypertension as a sustained elevation of arterial pressure above the normal range.

   You can then proceed to explain that the diastolic pressure is mostly used in the estimation of hypertension. This is because the systolic pressure normally fluctuates with changes in posture, exercise and emotion.

   Also explain that normal blood pressure for adults ranges between 100/60 and 140/90 mmHg and that hypertension is considered to be present if the diastolic pressure is consistently above 90 mmHg.

3

Prepare patient
- Explain and reassure the patient (worry will increase BP).
- Ensure rest for at least 15 minutes previously.
- Ensure that the patient is comfortable and relaxed.
- Ensure that his arm is well supported.
- Ensure that his clothing is out of the way of the cuff.

Prepare equipment
- Ensure that it is in working order.
- Turn the scale away from the patient so that he will not be unnecessarily worried.
- Check that the cuff is the correct size.

General preparation
- The surroundings should be quiet so that the nurse can hear accurately.
- Try to ensure that the same arm is used and that conditions do not vary.
- The arm should be held level with the patient's heart.

Take blood pressure
- Apply the cuff smoothly, ensuring that it covers the brachial artery.
- Take the systolic pressure accurately.
- Take the fourth and fifth sound for diastolic pressure (in line with ward policy).

Record blood pressure
- Complete the chart with date, time and readings.
- Compare it with previous readings.
- Make a note in the ward report, drawing particular attention to any changes.

4 - **Monday, 9 a.m.**
  Explain to Mr Westwood that his urine is to be saved for 24 hours from 10 a.m. Tell him that kidney disease can be the cause or effect of raised blood pressure, so the doctors want to measure his kidney function by looking at the content of a 24-hour urine specimen.

  Put the 24-hour collection bottle and a measuring jug in a tray in the sluice. Mark all three items clearly with Mr Westwood's name.
- **10 a.m.**
  Ask Mr Westwood to pass urine in the normal way and discard this specimen (which has been in the bladder before 10 a.m.). Show Mr Westwood the equipment and

ask him if he would mind collecting all his urine from now on and putting it into the bottle.

- **Tuesday, 10 a.m.**

  Ask Mr Westwood to pass the last specimen of urine to ensure that the collection has lasted for exactly 24 hours. Put it into the collection bottle. Ensure that the bottle label and the request form are filled in and put out for collection.

  Tell Mr Westwood that the collection has finished and that there is no longer any need to save his urine.

5 Essential hypertension means that his raised blood pressure is not caused by any other medical condition. Instead, the cause is largely unknown. However, there do seem to be some common risk factors:

- race (hypertension is more common in black people)
- stress
- obesity
- high dietary intake of salt and/or fats
- sedentary lifestyle
- family history of raised blood pressure
- use of tobacco

Because essential hypertension has no proven cause, it cannot be cured. This means that it is important that he realizes that he has a lifelong disease which needs continuous controlling. This means that he will need to take his tablets for the rest of his life and also try and reduce any of the above risk factors. (He will be given advice about this.) He must also ensure that he attends the clinic at regular intervals so that his blood pressure can be monitored.

6 Propranolol is a beta-blocker so you will first need to ask your junior colleague what she knows about the action of the sympathetic nervous system. She needs to know that sympathetic nerves convey their messages through release of noradrenaline and adrenaline.

You can then explain that drugs which affect the sympathetic nervous system are classified according to the receptors with which they interact. The sympathetic nervous system has two receptors—'alpha' and 'beta' receptors.

Beta-blocking drugs such as propranolol prevent the action of adrenaline and noradrenaline by occupying the beta-receptor site. Thus propranolol prevents the speeding up of the heart and the dilatation of blood vessels and bronchi. The side-effects are bradycardia and hypotension, due to the reduced cardiac output. Lightheadedness and visual disturbances are due to the vasoconstriction effect.

Prevention of bronchodilatation can cause bronchospasm. Central nervous system side-effects may also result, causing vivid dreams and feelings of disorientation.

7
- **Blood pressure recordings** Mr Westwood's blood pressure should be taken 4-hourly lying and standing to ensure postural hypotension does not occur.
- **Pulse** Mr Westwood's pulse should be taken 4-hourly to observe for bradycardia.
- **Observe** Mr Westwood for any signs of confusion. The night staff should report any disturbing dreams that prevent the patient from sleeping.
- **Ask** Mr Westwood if he has any new problems since commencing his drug treatment

8

Diet If Mr Westwood is overweight help him to choose a low-calorie reducing diet. Teach him the foods to avoid.
  Give him a low salt–low fat diet. Educate Mr Westwood about high fat and high salt foods to avoid.

Rest Help Mr Westwood to plan his day's activities to include a rest period. Find out what helps Mr Westwood to sleep and endeavour to provide the right environment, etc., to help him sleep at night.

Relaxation Explain all care and treatment beforehand. Give him time to express any fears or anxieties.

9
- **Dietary restriction** Sugary or starchy foods should be avoided (as weight reduction will reduce the strain on the heart). Salt intake should be restricted (as this reduces the work of the heart by reducing blood volume). Salty foods such as sausages, tinned meats, nuts and crisps should be avoided. Salt should not be added at the table.
- **Physical activity** A progressive programme of activity is beneficial when it is planned with your capability. (Lack of exercise results in a sluggish blood flow.)
- **Daily habits** Nicotine constricts blood vessels and raises blood pressure so it should be avoided. Coffee, tea and cola drinks all contain caffeine, which is also a vasoconstrictor. These should therefore only be taken in moderation.
- **Minimizing stress** Mr Westwood should try and identify

the stress factors in his life. Some of these might be avoided by altering his routine. Techniques that encourage muscular relaxation such as yoga, breathing exercises or meditation may be helpful in handling stress.

(The family should also be aware of the need to minimize stress by avoiding aggravating interpersonal situations arising in the home.)

10   The British Heart Foundation estimate that one in six adults suffers from hypertension. Studies in Scotland and England indicate that these figures could be higher as only about half of hypertensives have even been diagnosed.

Most heart attacks and strokes occur in patients with mild hypertension. Angina and heart failure are also common complications of hypertension.

Efficient reduction in blood pressure definitely prevents both heart attacks and strokes. Therefore, it seems important that the public is made aware of these facts and of the importance of having regular blood pressure checks.

Health education needs to inform the general public that maintenance of normal blood pressure can be helped by maintaining an ideal weight for the individual's sex, weight and height.

Salt can precipitate hypertension. Daily salt is provided by a usual diet and in cooking methods. There should be no need to add extra salt at the table.

Unsaturated fats, lean meats and grilling rather than frying foods will help to reduce the amount of saturated fats and cholesterol foods which are linked with the formation of atherosclerosis.

Exercise, as long as it is planned to suit the individual's capabilities, is beneficial. It seems to improve coronary circulation and lower blood cholesterol levels.

More emphasis should be given to the identification and reduction of stress in the individual's life. Too much stress can cause irritability, headaches, palpitations, etc., and certainly aggravates known hypertension.

1.3   Mrs Bates—a woman with bacterial endocarditis

Mrs Louise Bates, aged 35 years, is admitted to the ward with bacterial endocarditis. On admission she looks thin, pale and unwell and has a pyrexia of 38.5°C. She is very weak. Her husband, who is very anxious about her condition, says that he thought she had flu but that she had gradually become worse.

Mrs Bates is a housewife with two small children, aged 3 and 5 years. Her mother is staying at the family's home to look after the children while she is in hospital. Mr Bates is a computer programmer who works shifts.

Mrs Bates had rheumatic fever as a child but has always been comparatively well until this illness. She is to be nursed at rest. An intravenous cannula has been inserted and antibiotics prescribed, to be given every 6 hours for 4 weeks.

1   What specific information will be required from Mr and Mrs Bates on admission in order to plan Mrs Bates' care?

2   How would you explain Mrs Bates' condition to a junior colleague?

3   Explain the significance of the observations that will be carried out on Mrs Bates.

4   How can you help to allay Mr Bates' feelings of guilt and anxiety about his wife's condition?

5   Mrs Bates becomes anxious about her children missing her. How can you help to reassure her?

6   What actions should be taken to prevent potential phlebitis due to Mrs Bates' prolonged antibiotic therapy?

7   What information must be given to Mr and Mrs Bates when Mrs Bates is ready for discharge?

8   Describe the changing incidence of bacterial endocarditis.

1.3   Answers

1   Find out from Mrs Bates what problems she has as a result of her illness
   - Does she feel feverish? Is this at any particular time of day?
   - Does she have any pain? (Tender, raised lesions are sometimes found on the fingers and toes, called Osler's nodes.) Does she have her own way of relieving the pain?
   - Is she easily fatigued? What can she do without becoming overtired?
   - What is her appetite like? What does she like to eat and when? How much weight has she lost since she first felt ill?
   - Find out from Mr and Mrs Bates how much they understand about Mrs Bates' condition and its treatment
   - Endeavour to discover how Mrs Bates feels about her illness and its lengthy treatment
   - Ask about Mrs Bates' hobbies and interests; as she begins to feel better she could become bored and depressed with hospital.
   - What are Mr Bates' shifts? When is he able to visit? (Care can be avoided at these times whenever possible.)
   - Has Mrs Bates got any obvious infection sources? (Bad teeth? Skin lesions? Sore throat? Urinary infections?) These will need to be identified and treated to prevent further cardiac involvement.

2   Ask your junior colleague to draw a diagram of the heart, indicating the heart valves and the endocardium. This will give an idea of her present knowledge. Using her diagram (see Fig. 2) you can continue by explaining that endocarditis means an acute or subacute bacterial (or fungal) invasion of the lining of the heart.

   The pathogens may enter the body via the skin, respiratory, gastrointestinal or genitourinary tracts. Patients who have had congenital or rheumatic heart defects or open heart surgery are at most risk of such pathogens settling on the endocardium and, in particular, on the heart valves. The organisms multiply to set up vegetations. These vegetations may either reduce the lumen of the valves or prevent them from closing efficiently. Multiple emboli may be a complication of endocarditis as the vegetation can become dislodged from the valves and travel in the circulation.

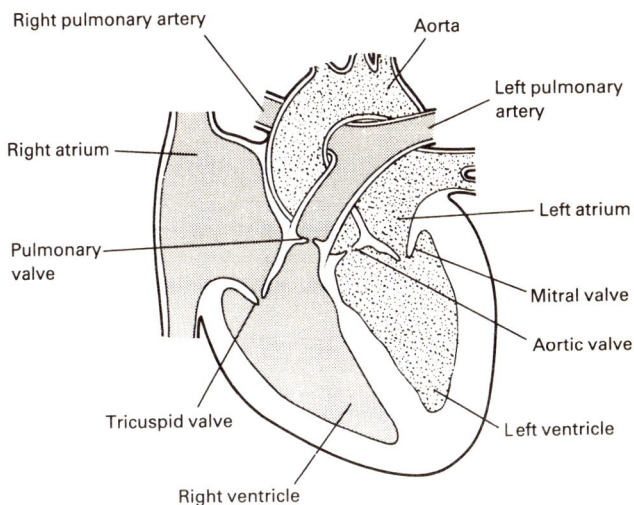

Fig. 2 Diagrammatic representation of the heart illustrating the heart valves and the endocardium.

3   The significance of Mrs Bates' observations lies in the detection of early signs of cardiac involvement, complications of bed rest, and emboli caused by dislodged vegetations.

Observations	Significance
Temperature	Continued pyrexia indicates that the source of infection has not been resolved.
Pulse	Irregularity and/or tachycardia indicate valvular damage.
Respirations	Dyspnoea on exertion may be a sign of heart failure. Dyspnoea and haemoptysis are indicative of a pulmonary embolus.
Pain	Acute abdominal pain may be due to a mesenteric embolus. Chest discomfort may result from heart failure. Abdominal discomfort may be caused by an enlarged spleen.

	Loin pain may be due to a deep vein thrombosis caused by immobility Excruciating pain in one leg accompanied by pallor, paraesthesia and cold indicates an embolus.
Urine testing	Haematuria is a sign of renal emboli.
Weight	Continued weight loss means that nursing actions, with regard to maintaining the patient's nutritional status, needs amendment.
Spontaneous movement	Any loss of power, consciousness or speech are indicative of a cerebral embolus.
Bowel pattern	Mrs Bates is pyrexial and anorexic and may easily become constipated.

4
- reassure Mr Bates that the onset of endocarditis is insidious and that there was no reason for him to realize the true problem
- spend time listening to his anxieties, answering questions, and reinforcing explanations
- encourage visits when he is not working, and involve in care as applicable. He might be able to bring his wife dietary treats to tempt her appetite
- allow the couple time alone together to discuss their feelings and anxieties

5
- encourage family contacts by letter and telephone calls
- allow short visits from the children
- allow afternoons out with her family as Mrs Bates progresses
- encourage Mrs Bates to talk about her children and suggest she gives them some belonging of hers to give them tangible evidence of her presence
- talk to Mr Bates. (He may be able to take photographs of the children to show her that they are enjoying themselves.)
- persuade Mrs Bates to talk to her mother about her worries

6
- cover the affected limb to avoid trauma
- ensure that the antibiotics are appropriately diluted before injection and are given over a safe length of time.
- remove covering of limb at least 4-hourly to observe for swelling, redness, or tenderness of the cannula site or the vein above. Report any signs of inflammation.
- ensure antibiotics are given with an aseptic technique.

- keep cannula site and dressing clean and dry.
- prior to insertion of antibiotics check the cannula for patency.

7   Mrs Bates must realize that the rheumatic fever she had as a child makes her liable to infections of the heart and that the endocarditis could re-occur. For this reason she needs to take preventative antibiotics when undergoing any procedure which could release bacteria into her blood circulation. Therefore, she should tell her dentist about her history of rheumatic fever, and she should remind any doctor who intends performing any minor surgery.

She must be told to seek advice from her general practitioner if she has persistent sore throats or skin infections, as this may be another indication for taking preventative antibiotics.

Mr and Mrs Bates should also realize that Mrs Bates has been acutely ill. She has been in hospital for some time, much of which was spent in bed. She cannot expect to be able to return to her usual activity immediately. It would be helpful if Mrs Bates' mother could stay for a little longer to help her. (If not, a home help could be arranged.) Mrs Bates should plan a daytime rest until she regains her strength.

Mrs Bates should recognize that it is important that she attends a follow-up clinic at regular intervals to monitor her heart function.

If the couple plan to have more children they would be advised to seek the advice of either their general practitioner or the clinic doctor first.

8   In recent years the incidence of bacterial endocarditis has changed. The relationship between rheumatic heart disease and bacterial endocarditis has always been marked, but now other patients have been found who are at risk from endocarditis.

An increased incidence of endocarditis is becoming apparent in patients who have had heart surgery, in drug addicts who use the intravenous route for their medication, and in those who have undergone invasive cardiac procedures such as cardiac catheterization and insertion of cardiac pacemakers.

Strict surgical asepsis is obviously essential for cardiac surgery, together with procedures to prevent this complication. Drug addicts should be warned of this added complication to their habit and advised about sterility of their equipment.

1.4   Mrs Williams—a woman who is undergoing surgery for varicose veins

Mrs Cathy Williams, aged 34 years, has been admitted for stripping and ligation of her varicose veins. Mrs Williams is married with two sons aged 10 and 14 years. She worked as a hairdresser in a salon near her home.

Her varicose veins have been present for some years. In the last couple of years she has suffered from fatigue, leg pains and cramp in her calf muscles.

Mrs Williams has a family history of varicose veins. Her mother was in this ward last year after knocking her leg, causing severe bleeding.

1   Describe the specific information required from Mrs Williams preoperatively, and her specific preparation for surgery.
2   Explain the anatomy and physiology of varicose veins to your junior colleague.
3   Describe the first aid treatment for bleeding varicose veins.
4   Mrs Williams asks you if her job has contributed to the presence of her varicose veins. How will you reply?
5   Mrs Williams says she feels a fraud for having such a small operation because she is ashamed of the appearance of her legs, when others in the ward are so ill. How can you reassure her?
6   Using a problem-solving approach plan Mrs Williams' care for the day after surgery.
7   Describe how Mrs Williams should be taught to apply her elastic bandages postoperatively.
8   Describe the advice Mrs Williams will require on her discharge from hospital 2 days after surgery.

1.4 Answers

1

Past medical history
- Has Mrs Williams been confined to bed (e.g. with flu) before admission?
- Has she had a feverish illness recently?
- Is her temperature raised on admission?

(Recent immobility and acute illness both increase the risk of deep vein thrombosis and are contraindications to varicose vein surgery.)

Menstrual history
- When was Mrs Williams' last menstruation?
- Is she pregnant?

(Because of the increased abdominal pressure during pregnancy, surgery is inadvisable at this time. In the period immediately before menstruation the leg vessels become full and heavy and varicose veins are more prominent, so avoid this time when operating.)

Contraceptive history
- Is Mrs Williams taking the contraceptive pill?
- If so, which one?

(While no connection between varicose veins and the contraceptive pill has been proven, it is advisable to discontinue its use during hospitalization because of the risk of deep vein thrombosis following vascular surgery. Anticoagulants are usually prescribed to patients who have been taking the contraceptive pill.)

Preparation
Shave from toe to groin, and the pubic area. Give the patient an explanation of the surgery. Three incisions will be made, one in the groin, one at the bend of the knee, and one in the inner surface of the foot, by the ankle. The affected veins are removed with a long probe inserted into these incisions ('stripping'). 'Ligating' refers to the stitching of the incisions at the end of the operation.

A crêpe bandage is then applied from groin to ankle before Mrs Williams returns to the ward.

Four to six hours after return she will be expected to get up and walk. Bed rest can be dangerous after this type of surgery, so it is important that the circulation in the leg is stimulated as soon as possible. At first the legs may feel clumsy and painful; medication can be given for the pain. The clumsy feeling soon wears off with exercise.

2 First check your junior colleague's present knowledge by asking her how blood in the leg veins is prevented from flowing backwards.

You can then explain that varicose veins result from defects in these venous valves. First, the proximal valves in the legs fail, increasing the column of blood that must be supported by the distal veins.

This increased pressure distends the veins, giving rise to a characteristic 'knot-like' appearance of varicose veins. This increased pressure may also cause rupture of the associated capillaries, producing petechial haemorrhages.

The cause of the valve failure is destruction of the vein walls, believed to result from man's upright posture (quadrupeds do not suffer from varicosities) and the consequent increased internal pressure in the leg veins.

The increased pressure is aggravated further by obesity, pregnancy and abdominal tumours. Sedentary jobs and lack of exercise also aggravate the condition by consistent stasis and pooling of blood in the legs.

3
- Reassure the patient.
- Lay the patient down and elevate the leg above the level of the heart.
- With a clean handkerchief, tea towel, etc., press firmly on the bleeding spot.
- Monitor the patient's condition by observing for shock— a weak, fast pulse; pale clammy skin; deeper respirations.
- If bleeding continues and/or the patient is severely shocked, send for an ambulance.

4 Tell Mrs Williams that the tendency towards varicose veins is inherited and that 80% of patients with varicose veins have inherited the tendency from parents and grandparents.

Prolonged standing has little to do with the formation of varicose veins. Indeed, it is better to have such a job, providing she does not stand still for long periods, than to have a sedentary life (see ans. 2).

5 You should reassure Mrs Williams that she is right to have surgery to her legs. Apart from the obvious cosmetic advantage, she will avoid the following complications of varicose veins:
- haemorrhage following damage to an affected vein
- ulceration following injury and infection to the area
- inflammation caused by extremes of temperature or trauma to the affected area

6

Problem	Aim	Nursing Care	Evaluation
Pain	To relieve Mrs Williams of pain so that she can take frequent walks	• Offer analgesia before Mrs Williams gets up and at 4–6-hourly intervals.	Patient able to walk freely without pain
Potential deep vein thrombosis	To encourage venous return by venous support and early mobility	• apply elastic bandage to legs from ankle to groin before patient gets up. • Encourage frequent 5/10-minute walks alternating with periods of rest in the chair, with legs elevated. • Observe bandage and reapply whenever it becomes loose. • Be alert for complaints of calf pain.	Patient mobilizing well Bandages applied correctly
Unable to bathe	To help patient to wash	• Offer bowl at bedside, or chair at the sink	Patient able to wash

7   Explain to Mrs Williams the importance of the bandages—
their firm resistance impedes the calf muscle from stretching
outwards. This pressure is transmitted to the deep veins of
the leg and helps to pump blood towards the heart, thus
preventing the formation of clots. It is therefore important

that the bandages are applied correctly and reapplied whenever they become loose.

As the bandage is elastic, it should not be stretched, but applied with constant pressure. It is not necessary to bandage the tip of the foot, which would make walking difficult, but bandaging should start over the instep. Bandage spirally from the the outer side of the foot inwards, passing the bandage from hand to hand. Overlap the previous turn by about three-quarters of an inch.

Mrs Williams can best be shown how to apply the bandages herself by a quick demonstration followed by a slower example accompanied by the above explanation. Then she should be allowed to do it herself with supervision.

She should be told to wear her compression bandages whenever she is out of bed for at least 2 weeks post-operatively. Then she can wear elastic stockings until checked in clinic after 6 weeks.

8   It is important to emphasize to Mrs Williams that her operation has only overcome her visible varicose veins. Her tendency to varicosities has not changed and she should make every effort to prevent further problems. She should:

- elevate her legs when sitting whenever possible
- avoid prolonged standing. She should walk about on the spot instead.
- avoid prolonged sitting. She should walk for at least 5 minutes every hour.
- wear elastic bandages for stockings initially. These should be washed daily and replaced when worn or loose.
- avoid constriction of the venous supply by tight girdles or corsets. She should also avoid constriction by sitting with her legs crossed or with the edge of the chair cutting into the backs of the legs.
- maintain a normal weight range and avoid obesity.

1.5 Mr Cannon—a man who has had a pulmonary embolus

Mr Max Cannon, aged 45 years, has been resting in bed at home for 3 weeks following a back injury at work. Suddenly, one afternoon, he awoke from a nap complaining of breathlessness and chest pain.

His wife called an ambulance and he has now arrived in the accident and emergency department.

1 As the admitting nurse, what immediate care would you carry out for Mr Cannon?

2 List, giving reasons, what necessary details will be required from Mrs Cannon once Mr Cannon has been cared for.

A pulmonary embolus is diagnosed and Mr Cannon is to be transferred to the acute medical ward. An i.v. cannula has been inserted and i.v. heparin 10 000 units has been prescribed 6-hourly. One oral dose of warfarin 40 mg has been prescribed.

3 List the responsibilities of the nurse accompanying Mr Cannon to the ward from the accident and emergency department.

4 How would you explain Mr Cannon's condition to your junior colleague?

5 Which one of the following situations is most likely to predispose to the development of a pulmonary embolus:
   (a) 50-year-old man 3 days after a myocardial infarction?
   (b) 25-year-old male in traction for 5 weeks for a fractured femur?
   (c) 35-year-old woman after 2 weeks with a broken leg in plaster?
   (d) 20-year-old obese female one day after a caesarian section?

6 Explain why Mr Cannon has been prescribed both heparin and warfarin.

7 What nursing actions must be planned to monitor any side-effects of Mr Cannon's anticoagulant therapy?

8 Describe Mr Cannon's treatment at each level of mobility during his stay in hospital.
9 What advice should Mr Cannon be given before discharge?
10 Describe the prevention of vascular thrombosis.

1.5 Answers

1 • Reassure Mr and Mrs Cannon.
  • Help the ambulancemen to *lift* Mr Cannon onto the accident department trolley.
  • Place him in an upright position.
  • Provide oxygen 24% via a venti-mask. Explain to Mr Cannon that this is to help his breathing.
  • Take note of the ambulancemen's history and observations.
  • Tell Mr Cannon that the doctor will soon be there to see him.
  • Take and record a set of observations from Mr Cannon (temperature, pulse, respirations, blood pressure).

2 • Full name and address (to ensure that Mr Cannon is correctly identified and to facilitate the finding of any hospital notes)
  • Birth-date (to help with disease indexing)
  • Religion (to appreciate any special associated needs)
  • Nationality (to appreciate cultural needs)
  • General practitioner (to inform him of the admission and the details of his treatment on discharge)
  • Allergies (to prevent any mishaps)
  • Past medical history (to prevent complications resulting from ignoring other conditions, e.g. diabetes) and any medication
  • Symptoms (to discover if there are any other features of this illness, e.g. haemoptysis)
  • Her address and telephone number so that she can be contacted

3 • To explain to Mr and Mrs Cannon what is happening
  • To ensure that she has Mr Cannon's charts, notes, X-rays and property on the trolley
  • To check that the oxygen and portable suction on the trolley are functioning
  • To stay at the head of the trolley during transportation
  • To reassure the patient on the journey
    On arrival at the ward:
  • To find Mrs Cannon a seat
  • To help the porter to lift Mr Cannon into bed and ensure that he is comfortable
  • To introduce Mr and Mrs Cannon to the receiving nurse-in-charge (or the allocated nurse); to explain Mr Cannon's condition at the time, any treatment given in the accident

department, and any special instructions regarding care; and to pass on his notes and X-rays.
- To give Mr Cannon's property to the ward nurse and to ensure that she signs for it.

4   To assess her present knowledge, you should first ask your junior colleague to define pulmonary embolus. She should define it as an obstruction in the pulmonary circulation.

You can then explain that the obstruction is usually caused by a dislodged thrombus, but that it can be caused by any foreign matter (e.g. fat embolism, air embolism, amniotic fluid embolism, tumour embolism).

In Mr Cannon's case his prolonged bed rest has resulted in venous stasis. This stagnation of the circulation has caused clotting in the deep veins of the legs. Deep vein thrombosis is often silent and only becomes apparent in retrospect when a piece of thrombus becomes dislodged to travel in the circulation and cause a pulmonary embolus.

The dislodged thrombus travels easily through the venous circulation and the right side of the heart. It passes into the pulmonary artery but then occludes one of the subdivisions of this artery. Infarction occurs in the area of lung supplied by the occluded vessel.

If the occluded blood vessel is large and the area of infarction is extensive, sudden death may occur. If the occluded area is small, as in Mr Cannon's case, the pulmonary infarction results in breathlessness and chest pain.

5   (b). All these patients are at risk of venous stasis and resultant thrombosis and embolism. However, the patient on traction is most at risk because of his long period of immobilization.

6   Heparin and warfarin are both anticoagulants which are given to prevent the extension of the thrombus in the pulmonary circulation and also to prevent the development of further thrombi in the leg veins.

Warfarin takes about 48 hours to act, so heparin must be given to cover this period of time. Intravenous heparin acts almost immediately but only lasts for 6–8 hours, so it needs to be given at least four times daily.

Heparin can be given for 48 hours and discontinued when the action of warfarin has commenced. The patient can continue on oral warfarin, the dosage of which depends on daily prothrombin times.

7   - Daily inspection of urine for haematuria
- Inspection of stools for malaena

- Checks to ensure that Mr Cannon does not experience excessive bleeding from cuts or nose bleeds
- Observation of Mr Cannon for bruising
- Inspection of any vomit for 'coffee grounds' or obvious blood

8 Initially, bed rest is essential to prevent further embolization. However, it is important to reposition and exercise Mr Cannon's legs and to teach him deep breathing exercises to prevent venous stasis and further clotting problems.

Once Mr Cannon's prothrombin time is stable at a therapeutic level ($2\frac{1}{2}$ times the normal control of 35–45 seconds) he can begin to remobilize (providing his back injury is also stable). Antiembolism stockings should be applied and Mr Cannon should be advised to avoid sudden exertion and leg movements. Such activities could initiate a thrombus to dislodge. He should also be careful not to knock his leg for the same reason.

9

To continue warfarin
- Always take it as prescribed.
- Do not run out of it.
- Attend the haematology clinic weekly for blood tests to monitor the effectiveness of the drug.
- Be prepared to alter the dosage according to results of the blood test.

To watch for bleeding (a side-effect of warfarin)
- Check stools for tarry appearance or obvious blood.
- Check urine for blood.
- If either of above occur, go to general practitioner.
- Expect a longer bleed if trauma occurs (when shaving for example).

To inform others of anticoagulant therapy
- Carry a card giving details of medication.
- Tell dentist, chiropodist, etc., of this treatment.

To avoid potentiating or counteracting the effect of warfarin
- Do not take aspirin (or other medicines containing aspirin).
- Do not take alcohol in excess.
- Remind your general practitioner if other medication is prescribed.

(A booklet can be given to Mr Cannon to consolidate this advice.)

10   In order to prevent this cause of pulmonary embolus it is necessary to consider the following causes of thrombus formation:

- **Hypercoaguability of blood (e.g. polycythaemia)** Little can be done to reduce thrombus formation in this situation.

- **Trauma to vessel walls** Damage to vessel walls can be avoided by changing the patient's body position. Such alterations in position prevent venous distension and pooling of blood in dependent areas. Healthy people automatically alter their position every half-hour at least. Therefore, it is important to reposition patients who cannot move themselves at least 2-hourly.

  Patients who are more mobile must be advised about the dangers of lying in one position for too long. They should also be warned not to sit or lie with their legs crossed, which puts undue pressure on the leg veins.

- **Venous status** In patients confined to bed, immobility decreases blood flow by about 50% because of the decreased muscle tone. Immobility also causes generalized dilatation of blood vessels due to increased activity of the parasympathetic nervous system. This vasodilatation leads to pooling of blood in dependent areas.

  Early ambulation should be encouraged after surgery. Patients confined to bed should be taught leg exercises and deep breathing exercises to encourage venous return. Antiembolism stockings may also be used. However, it is essential that the patient is taught the reason for these preventive measures if he is to cooperate.

  Passive exercises and physiotherapy should be performed for patients who are unable to move for themselves.

2 Care of the Patient with an Endocrine Disorder

2.1   Mrs Spencer—an adult having an adrenalectomy

Mrs Ruth Spencer, aged 44 years, was diagnosed as having carcinoma of the breast 2 years ago when she had a mastectomy and radiotherapy. She has now relapsed and doctors have decided to perform an adrenalectomy in order to induce regression of the tumour.

Mrs Spencer is married and her husband has accompanied her to the hospital. During the admission assessment it becomes evident that neither of them really understands why the operation is being done or its implications.

1   What response would you make when Mr and Mrs Spencer ask you to explain the operation and its implications?
2   Explain, giving reasons, the specific pre-operative care Mrs Spencer will require.

Mrs Spencer goes to theatre 4 days after admission. She returns to the ward with an intravenous infusion in situ.

3   With reference to altered physiology, how would you explain the significance of Mrs Spencer's post-operative observations to the junior nurse assigned to work with you?
4   Giving reasons, what nursing actions should be implemented in order to ensure that Mrs Spencer mobilizes safely post-operatively?

Mrs Spencer is commenced on hydrocortisone and fludrocortisone during surgery. The dosage is adjusted according to Mrs Spencer's clinical state and gradually reduced to a maintenance dose.

5   What may be the early signs of side-effects of the steroids for which the nurse must be observant?

Ten days post-operatively Mrs Spencer's wound has healed well and the sutures are ready for removal.

6 What would you teach the junior nurse about the principles of removing sutures?
7 What should Mr and Mrs Spencer be taught about her medication in preparation for discharge?
8 What other information and advice should Mrs Spencer be given on discharge?

2.1   Answers

1   • It is important to find out first what they have already been told by the doctor and then to ascertain their level of understanding.
   • Use a diagram to show them the position of the adrenal glands.
   • Explain that in some cases of breast cancer, the causes seem to be related to a high level of certain hormones, mainly oestrogen.
   • Explain the functions of oestrogen.
   • As the cancer cells are hormone-dependent, removing the hormone should produce a remission. Oestrogen is produced in the ovaries (which were removed during her previous surgery) and in the adrenal glands. Therefore, removal of the glands will stop the production of oestrogens completely.
   • The adrenal glands also secrete other hormones which are essential to life, so Mrs Spencer will have to take hormone replacement therapy for the rest of her life, even if she feels well.

2

Specific pre-operative care	Reasons
Recording of blood pressure to serve as a comparison post-operatively	One potential problem post-operatively is hypotension, so it is important to know Mrs Spencer's normal blood pressure.
Education of patient with regard to deep breathing and coughing	Post-operatively, respirations may tend to be shallow because the incision is so close to the diaphragm.
Shaving of nipple to pubis, and cleansing	This depends on the surgeon's wishes and reduces the incidence of post-operative infection.
Passage of a nasogastric tube	This prevents post-operative vomiting and abdominal distension.
Assisting the doctor with taking blood and siting intravenous infusion	Infusion is commenced to administer hydrocortisone to prevent adrenal insufficiency.

Care and maintenance of infusion	This ensures that hydrocortisone is administered slowly and as prescribed.

3

Observations	Significance/Altered physiology	
Blood pressure	Low blood pressure	These features may indicate corticoid insufficiency or lack of aldosterone. Will cause an increased excretion of sodium and water leading to lowered blood volume.
Pulse	Tachycardia	
Respirations	Dyspnoea	
	Low blood pressure Tachycardia	These features could indicate haemorrhage.
Temperature	Raised temperature may indicate acute corticoid insufficiency.	
Fluid intake and output chart	All fluid intake and output must be measured and charted. Any imbalance must be reported immediately. An increase in urine output could indicate corticoid insufficiency, as may vomiting. Mrs Spencer may become dehydrated.	
General condition	Increased weakness, lethargy and confusion are indicative of a high serum potassium which is a result of insufficient aldosterone. Headache, nausea, vomiting and twitching are indicative of a low serum sodium.	

4   Postoperatively there is a danger of hypotension due to lack of aldosterone, which is usually secreted from the adrenal cortex. Excess sodium will be excreted as well as water, and blood volume and therefore blood pressure falls. Until maintenance dosages of steroids are established the blood pressure will tend to fluctuate. The patient will not be able to cope with maintaining blood when changing position (standing or sitting up from a lying position). For this reason, the following nursing actions should be taken:

- Nurse Mrs Spencer flat in the initial post-operative period. Change position slowly.
- Ensure that Mrs Spencer remains in bed and check her blood pressure before mobilizing.
- Raise the head of the bed and check her blood pressure before mobilizing.
- Stay with Mrs Spencer when she is eventually permitted to get up.
- Check her blood pressure every 15 minutes initially; if there is a significant fall in blood pressure, Mrs Spencer should be returned to bed and kept flat.

5   The steroids Mrs Spencer has been prescribed are 'replacement therapy'. That is they are intended to meet a physiological need. There should be no side-effects in replacement therapy as the dosages are lower than in other treatment. If side-effects do occur, they indicate overdosage and should be reported immediately.

Early signs of side-effects are:
- restlessness, swings in mood and euphoria
- muscle wasting/weakness due to excessive protein breakdown
- oedema caused by sodium and water retention
- 'moon face'—characteristic rounding of the face—caused by increased deposition of fat
- growth of hair on the face

6
- The wound must be well healed.
- Aseptic technique must be used.
- Scissors or stitch cutters may be used.
- No suture material above the skin should be allowed to pass through the subcutaneous layer after the stitch has been cut.
- The suture should be removed towards the incision line.
- Alternate sutures should be removed initially in case the wound gapes.
- The wound should be cleansed if necessary.

7   Mrs Spencer must continue to take the drugs at all times. Both she and Mr Spencer must realize that to stop taking the drug could have serious consequences. A simple explanation should be given.
- Mrs Spencer must carry a corticosteroid card with her at all times and/or wear a medical alert bracelet/necklace to inform others that she is taking steroids should an illness/accident necessitate emergency treatment.
- Mrs Spencer should take the drugs at the prescribed times and after meals (to reduce possible gastric irritation).

- She should take no other medicines without permission from her physician.
- They must understand that any stressful situations or illness will increase her need for steroids. Mrs Spencer should therefore avoid any emotional disturbances and worry as much as possible, and avoid people with colds and other illnesses. In the event of any illness, fainting or sudden weakness, she should seek medical attention. Mr and Mrs Spencer may be taught how to give intramuscular injections of hydrocortisone in emergencies.
- All instructions should be given in written form.

8
- The importance of adequate and regular rest
- To avoid cold/stress
- To pay attention to diet, which should be high protein and high carbohydrate with specified amounts of sodium. Meals should be regular with a bedtime snack to maintain normal blood sugar level, and a dietician should be involved.
- To resume activities slowly. It may take several months to adjust hormonal replacement satisfactorily.
- The importance of attending outpatient's appointments. The date of the first appointment should be provided.
- How to contact help if needed, and the telephone number of the ward (for advice).

2.2 Nicola Barnes—an adolescent with diabetes mellitus

Nicola Barnes, aged 15 years, is admitted to the ward for restabilization of her diabetes. Nicola was diagnosed as having diabetes mellitus when she was 8-years-old. She has been well until recently, when she has had difficulty in controlling her blood sugar level. Nicola lives at home with her mother who is a teacher, her father who is a bank manager, and her two younger brothers. She attends the local grammar school and is to take her O levels in 6 months time. Her hobbies are swimming and horse riding, and she belongs to the local Guide Company.

On admission Nicola's blood sugar level is raised and she is drowsy, vomiting and slightly dehydrated.

1 What information would you elicit from Nicola and her parents during your initial assessment?

2 Using a problem-solving approach identify Nicola's needs and problems in relation to her condition on admission, and explain, giving reasons, the nursing actions you would instigate.

3 List the possible reasons for Nicola's unstable blood sugar level.

4 With reference to anatomy and physiology explain the effects that hyperglycaemia may have on Nicola.

5 List the observations you would make of Nicola during her stay and explain the significance of these observations and the role they play in evaluation of care.

6 What should Nicola and her parents have been taught regarding insulin and its administration?

7 According to recent literature what are the principles of dietary management for diabetic patients?

Nicola complains of a headache and is found to be pale and sweating 48 hours following admission.

8 With reference to anatomy and physiology explain what is happening to Nicola.

9   What may be the cause of this attack and what actions
    should the nurse take?

Nicola is ready for discharge after 4 days. She and her parents have
been told about the complications of poor diabetic control in the past
but need to have some points reiterated.

---

10   List at least four long-term complications of diabetes.
11   What information and advice should Nicola and her parents
     be given regarding:
     (a)   periods of illness
     (b)   her forthcoming exams and future career
     (c)   activities

2.2   Answers

1   • Name, age, address and telephone number of parents for contact
     • Base-line observations of temperature, pulse, respirations, blood pressure and level of consciousness; any signs of a decreasing level of consciousness or infection
     • Weight; initial urine test for glucose and ketones; capillary blood glucose (compare results with those Nicola recorded before admission); information regarding present dosage/type of insulin and details of diet
     • The degree to which Nicola manages her own condition
     • The normal daily routine regarding activities of living, e.g. hygiene, sleep, elimination, exercise, hobbies, educational needs, menstruation
     • Any previous problems with control of blood sugar level

2

Need/problem	Nursing action	Rationale
Drowsiness and potential coma due to high blood sugar	• Administer insulin as prescribed.	Reduces blood sugar level
	• Maintain safe environment.	May injure herself
	• Monitor level of consciousness.	To detect deterioration
	• Ensure patent airway.	May inhale vomit if drowsy
Vomiting	• Provide vomit bowl (and privacy!)	
	• Wash hands and face.	To ensure comfort
	• Ensure mouth care.	
	• Ensure that suction equipment is available.	
Dehydration	• Encourage fluids.	Negative fluid balance would indicate the need for an intravenous infusion. Infusion would rehydrate Nicola.
	• Record fluid balance.	
	• Ensure care of intravenous infusion if in situ.	

Fear	• Explain what is happening to Nicola and her parents. • Be calm and efficient. • Invite and answer questions.	An informed patient and relative will be more relaxed.

3 • Pubertal growth and physical changes
   • Emotional instability—conflict with parents, rebellion against authority, and a need to be like her peers
   • Failure to take adequate insulin
   • Overeating
   • Infections

4 Food is taken in as usual and glucose enters the blood. As there is no insulin the cells are unable to utilize the glucose. The effects of this are as follows:
   • The level of glucose in the blood rises—hyperglycaemia.
   • Eventually the level of glucose passes the renal threshold and glucose is excreted in the urine—glycosuria.
   • Glycosuria increases the osmotic pressure of urine within the tubules and water is not reabsorbed, polyuria and dehydration.
   • The body tries to compensate for polyuria by increasing fluid intake, resulting in polydipsia.
   • As glucose is not able to be utilized, fatigue and lethargy result.
   • The body tries in vain to gain energy by converting proteins and fats to glucose, which aggravates the hyperglycaemia.
   • The use of body proteins results in general tiredness, weight loss and loss of muscle bulk.
   • The use of body fats results in weight loss and accumulation of the products of fat metabolism (vomiting, acidotic breath, ketonuria, confusion), which, in turn, results in coma.

5

Observation	Significance and role in evaluation of care
Level of consciousness	• To monitor signs of increasing/decreasing hyperglycaemia. If care is effective Nicola should become less drowsy and fully orientated.

	• To monitor signs of hypoglycaemia, i.e. sudden loss of consciousness.
Temperature, pulse and blood pressure	To detect infection, hyperglycaemia (weak rapid pulse) and hypotension. Return of these to normal indicates effective management.
Respirations	To detect hyperglycaemia (deep sighing respirations as a result of acidosis). Normal respirations indicate effective care.
Fluid intake and output chart	Monitor for decreasing urine output. Decreasing thirst indicates effective management of hyperglycaemia. Observe any vomiting—reduction in vomiting indicates reduced acidosis.
Weight	Weight gain indicates improved hydration and effective use of glucose.
Urinalysis (ketones + glucose 4-hourly initially)	Urine should ideally be free of ketones with no glucose or a trace only. An increase in either ketones or glucose would indicate the need for more insulin.
Capillary blood glucose (BM sticks/ dextrostix)	The normal level is 4–10 mmol/litre. This is a more precise method of determining blood sugar levels than urine testing. The time of the test in relation to meals must be taken into consideration.
Attitude of both Nicola and her parents to her condition	This reflects Nicola's increasing/ decreasing interest in control of her diabetes and the effectiveness of psychological support.

6   • Action of insulin
   • Different types of insulin, duration of action, and side-effects
   • Storage of insulin
   • Equipment—how to obtain it, store it and sterilize it
   • How to draw up the insulin and mix insulins
   • Sites for injection and importance of varying sites
   • How to give the injection

- How to dispose of needles and syringes
- How to vary the dose of insulin according to needs
7 - Calorie intake should be tailored to suit individual needs.
- The carbohydrate content of the diet should be at least 50% of the total calorie intake, and should be in the polysaccharide form (e.g. bread, potatoes) where absorption is slower and steadier.
- High-fibre carbohydrates are preferred because they slow absorption and help to control calorie intake.
- Rapidly absorbed carbohydrates should be avoided.
- Fats should comprise no more than 35% of the total calorie intake.
- Diabetic foods must be used with care.
- The timing of carbohydrate intake is important.
- Salt intake should be kept to a minimum.

References

British Diabetic Association (1982) *Dietary Recommendations for Diabetics for the 1980s*

Anderson, JW (1981) *Diabetics: A Practical New Guide to Healthy Living*. London: Martin Dunitz.

8 The blood sugar level has fallen below 4 mmol/litre. Brain cells are very dependent on a constant supply of glucose, so any deprivation may impair cerebral activity leading to dizziness, lability of mood, convulsions and coma.

A low blood sugar level stimulates sympathetic nervous system activity leading to palpitations, weakness, sweating and hunger.

9 **Causes**
- Controlled hyperglycaemic attack
- Overdose of insulin
- Low dietary intake of glucose
- Increased exercise/stress levels

Nursing actions
- Maintenance of airway if unconscious
- Administration of glucose or glucagon—oral/i.m./i.v. depending upon level of consciousness
- Monitoring of conscious levels and vital signs
- Test and chart blood glucose levels

10 - Peripheral neuritis
- Retinopathy, cataracts
- Renal disease
- Atherosclerosis
  1 Hypertension
  2 Myocardial infarction

 3 Cerebrovascular accident
 4 Intermittent claudication leading to gangrene
 • Varicose ulcers

11 (a) Nicola must take her usual dose of insulin, she should test her urine frequently, she should try to take her usual amount of carbohydrate, and the doctor should be informed. If urine tests show sugar and ketones, insulin dosage may need to be increased. Nicola must drink plenty of fluids.

(b) As glucose is used up faster during times of stress, Nicola should take extra glucose before an exam. Insulin dosage should remain as usual. Careers that have a regular routine offer an advantage over those that do not, but a diabetic who is well controlled may follow any career with two exceptions: driving heavy goods/passenger vehicles, and the armed forces. She should be honest about her condition.

(c) Exercise is an important method of keeping the blood sugar level as near to normal as possible. There are very few things Nicola cannot do, but rock climbing and sub-aqua swimming are not advised. She should have company when walking far from help and avoid swimming far out of her depth when alone. If necessary she should take extra glucose before exercise.

2.3 Mrs Armstrong—a woman with myxoedema

Mrs Sarah Armstrong, aged 52 years, is married with two grown-up children, both of whom have left school. Her husband is a college lecturer and Mrs Armstrong works part-time at the local hospital as a ward clerk. Several weeks ago Mrs Armstrong visited her general practitioner with her husband. Her family had been anxious about her health for some time, noticing that she had become increasingly lethargic and unsteady on her feet. The family had to persuade Mrs Armstrong to visit the doctor as she was disinclined to seek advice.

On examination the general practitioner found Mrs Armstrong to have bradycardia and a subnormal temperature (35.6°C). Mrs Armstrong complained of being constipated and of having lost her sense of taste and smell. She was gaining weight in spite of a decreased appetite. She had the characteristic appearance of a patient suffering from advanced hypothyroidism. Mrs Armstrong was referred to a consultant physician who, suspecting hypothyroidism, arranged for her to be admitted to the ward for investigations and treatment.

1 What would be the significance of the information the nurse should gain during the initial nursing assessment of Mrs Armstrong?
2 How would you explain to a junior colleague:
   (a) how the thyroid hormones are manufactured and the role that iodine plays?
   (b) how the production of thyroid hormone is controlled?
   (c) Mrs Armstrong's altered appearance?
3 Describe the care Mrs Armstrong will require during a radioactive iodine uptake test.

Following investigations the doctor confirms hypothyroidism and Mrs Armstrong is prescribed thyroxine replacement therapy. Mrs Armstrong is to remain in hospital until a maintenance dose is established.

4 List the symptoms that would lead the nurse to suspect an overdose of thryoxine.

5   Following a talk with Mrs Armstrong one of the nursing
    goals identified is for her to have her bowels open every
    other day by the time she goes home. Giving reasons, state
    the possible nursing actions to help her achieve this goal.
6   Identify the other problems (potential or actual) that
    Mrs Armstrong may have.

Mrs Armstrong's family visit her daily and are very keen to participate
in her care. They ask how they can best help and what the future may
hold.

---

7   What advice would you give Mrs Armstrong and her family
    in order that they may continue her care at home?
8   How can the effectiveness of Mrs Armstrong's care be evalu-
    ated when she is ready for discharge?

2.3   Answers

1

Information	Significance
Baseline observations of pulse, blood pressure and temperature	This gives an idea as to the degree of dysfunction of the thyroid gland, and enables a judgement to be made regarding improvement.
Present weight/normal weight	This gives the degree of weight gain and acts as a baseline for deciding dietary needs.
Normal elimination pattern when healthy and at present	This gives an idea of the target to be achieved and the degree of constipation.
Normal dietary intake	This enables adjustments to be made where needed.
Usual sleep pattern	This gives a baseline on which to monitor improvement.
Actions taken to keep warm	This enables appropriate nursing actions to be implemented
Hobbies, activities and degree of activity when well	This gives the normal level of activity and the degree to which dysfunction of the gland is affecting Mrs Armstrong.
Normal routine	This enables normal routine to be followed where possible.

Much of this information may have to be gained from the family to gain a baseline.

2   (a)   There are two main thyroid hormones: thyroxine (T_4) and triiodothyronine (T_3). The thyroid hormones are formed by the combination of the amino acid, tyrosine, and iodine.

The tyrosine combines with one or two atoms of iodine initially to form two compounds—monoiodotyrosine and diiodotyrosine.

Under the influence of an enzyme three compounds combine to form T_3 and T_4.

The hormones are stored, loosely coupled with a protein (thyroglobulin) in the thyroid gland until required.

A third hormone is manufactured in the thyroid gland called calcitonin.

(b)   The hypothalamus determines the sensitivity of the pituitary gland by producing thyrotrophin-releasing hormone (TRH), which acts on the pituitary gland. The anterior lobe of the pituitary gland is stimulated by a fall in T_4 and T_3 levels, which is controlled by the thyroid-stimulating hormone (TSH). This acts on the thyroid gland which, in turn, acts on T_4 and T_3.

(c)   The nurse should do the following:

- Ask the student what she already knows.
- Recap on the normal physiology of the thyroid gland and the functions of thyroxine.
- Explain the following features, which are caused by reduced thyroxine:
  1 General reduction in metabolic rate
  2 Retention of fluid in body tissues
  3 Abnormal deposition of a jelly-like substance (mucin), which occurs in subcutaneous tissues
- Explain that the following characteristics may be obvious:
  1 Dry, thick skin
  2 Sparse, dry hair and thin eyebrows
  3 Puffy face
  4 Podgy hands and fingers
  5 Enlarged lips and tongue
  6 Yellow tinged skin

3   Mrs Armstrong will first require an

- explanation of the procedure. She should be told that it is a very simple and quick procedure.
- The nurse should ensure that she realizes that the radio-active test is entirely safe and will have no harmful effects.
- Mrs Armstrong will then be asked to take a small drink via a straw; this contains the radioactive iodine solution.
- There is no need to shield the staff or patients.
- Special precautions are only required if Mrs Armstrong vomits following the drink. It should be contained but not disposed of without seeking advice from the radiation safety officer.
- The nurse should explain that a Geiger counter will be held over her neck to count the uptake of the iodine. Counting is usually done after 4 hours and 24 hours.
- The radioactive iodine will be excreted in the urine over the next few days.

4   • Rapid pulse rate

- Palpitations
- Restlessness/hyperactivity
- Insomnia
- Diarrhoea

5

Nursing action	Rationale
Encourage fluid intake—approximately 2 litres daily.	This helps to make stools softer by increasing the water content.
Encourage fresh fruit and a high fibre diet.	This adds bulk to the stool and speeds up the passage of faeces.
Establish a regular time for defecation, e.g. after breakfast.	This enables the individual to set aside a time to respond to stimuli.
Teach her abdominal exercises.	This strengthens the abdominal muscles and aids defecation.
Encourage normal exercise.	This increases/stimulates peristalsis.
Administer laxatives and enemas as prescribed.	This swells the faeces and provides bulk which stimulates peristalsis. It also softens the stools.

6
- Dry skin and hair
- Potential pressure sores
- Decreased tolerance to cold
- Weight gain
- Possible distress at altered appearance
- Mental and physical sluggishness
- Myxoedema madness

7 Replacement therapy must be continued indefinitely—Mrs Armstrong may want to stop taking the thyroxine when she feels well. She will need to be seen regularly as some adjustment of the dosage may be needed from time to time.

No change will be noticed in her condition for about 10 days when the drug takes effect. Indications of improvement should be pointed out to reassure the family that the condition is reversible. It should also be explained that Mrs Armstrong may not feel completely well again for some months. Relatives must be patient and tolerant of her slowness. She must be encouraged and given time to complete responses and activities. The care being given in hospital should be explained and the family included in drawing up the care plan.

8
- Pulse rate and temperature should begin to rise to near normal levels.
- There should be no reaction to therapy.
- There should be no development of pressure sores.
- The skin should become more supple.
- Mrs Armstrong should become a little less lethargic and more interested in her condition.
- She should understand the purpose of her therapy and future prognosis.
- The output chart should show bowel movement every other day.
- The family should understand the care that Mrs Armstrong will require
- She should understand her medication.

2.4   Mrs Watson—a woman with thyrotoxicosis

Mrs Watson, aged 32 years, is married with no children. She is a buyer for a large department store and her husband is an architect.

A year ago Mrs Watson had major spinal surgery. She recovered well but 6 months later she was encouraged to visit her general practitioner by her husband. He described her as being extremely anxious and nervous and she admitted to feeling constantly on 'the brink of disaster'. She was aware of her heart and her pulse beating and she was losing weight in spite of a good appetite. She also complained of excessive sweating and an intolerance to warm weather.

Her general practitioner referred her to a consultant physician who diagnosed thyrotoxicosis. Mrs Watson has been admitted to the ward for a partial thyroidectomy. In preparation for surgery she has been taking carbimazole for the past 12 weeks. One week before surgery this was discontinued and potassium iodide was commenced.

1   What effects may carbimazole have and what specific instructions should Mrs Watson have been given regarding this treatment?

2   Both Mrs Watson and her husband are concerned about the operation and her future health. What information and advice can they be given to reduce their anxiety?

3   With reference to altered physiology explain the problems Mrs Watson has presented with. List four other possible effects of hyperthyroidism.

4   Identify, giving reasons, the specific physical preparation Mrs Watson will require before theatre.

Mrs Watson returns from theatre having regained consciousness in the recovery ward. She has an intravenous infusion in progress and a redivac wound drain in situ. Morphine has been prescribed for pain.

5   With reference to altered anatomy and physiology explain the specific potential post-operative complications of thyroidectomy.

6   Explain the significance of Mrs Watson's post-operative observations for the first 48 hours after surgery.

7   Why is it important that Mrs Watson's post-operative analgesia is given regularly? How can nursing care be planned so as to minimize pain and discomfort?

Five days later Mrs Watson is taking normal diet. Her wound has healed well and the sutures have been removed. She is ready for discharge.

---

8   What information and advice should Mrs Watson be given prior to her discharge?

2.4   Answers

1   Carbimazole prevents the uptake of iodine by the thyroid gland. It may increase thyroid size and vascularity and is therefore stopped before surgery.

   Side-effects of carbimazole are rashes, fever, dermatitis and agranulocytosis.

   Mrs Watson should have been told to report promptly any sore throat, fever, rash or swollen neck glands. The drug must be taken regularly and at the hours suggested. Slight enlargement of the thyroid gland is to be expected.

2   The operation can be explained with the aid of a diagram.

   Mrs Watson should be informed that the scar will become barely perceptible within a few months of the operation. In the interval a scarf or necklace will conceal it.

   The symptoms to expect post-operatively—sore throat, difficulty in swallowing, and wound drain—should also be explained. Pain will be well controlled. She will have an intravenous infusion which will maintain her fluid intake until she begins to drink again.

   Mrs Watson should be told how long she is likely to be in hospital and it should be explained that, although her neck will be stiff at first, she should soon be able to move her head freely.

   Her future health should be good, but regular check-ups will be carried out.

   Mr Watson should be informed about visiting times and the time of operation and how long it is likely to take. He should be given the ward telephone number.

   They should both be encouraged to ask questions and given time to talk about their fears and worries.

3

Mrs Watson's problem	Altered physiology
Loss of weight	Increased metabolic rate
Intolerance of heat	Increased heat production in body
Excessive sweating	Increased activity of glands
Increased pulse rate	Increased metabolic demands and the effects of thyroxine on the sympathetic nervous system

| Palpitations | Increased heart rate and overworked heart due to increased blood circulation |
| Swings of mood, nervousness | Increased metabolic rate and its effect on nerve stability |

Other possible effects of hyperthyroidism
- Fine tremor of hands
- Exophthalmos
- Goitre
- Shortness of breath on exertion
- Lowered diastolic blood pressure
- Diarrhoea
- Menstrual disorders

4

Pre-operative preparation	Rationale
A restful environment in a well-ventilated room	To prevent unnecessary disturbance which may aggravate nervousness and excitability
Monitoring of pulse rate, especially sleeping pulse, although this is sometimes difficult to do	To ensure that the patient is in a euthyroid state for operation. Increasing pulse rate may indicate overactivity of the thyroid gland and the operation may have to be cancelled.
Blood tests for levels of T_3 and T_4	To monitor the degree of activity of the thyroid gland
Examination by ear, nose and throat surgeon	To check that both vocal cords are functioning well before surgery
Electrocardiogram	To obtain information about cardiac status
Administration of potassium iodide (Lugol's solution)	To reduce the size and vascularity of the thyroid gland and lessen the risk of haemorrhage
Thorough cleansing of neck, upper shoulders and chest	To reduce the possibility of infection and improve wound healing (dependent on the surgeon)
Tying up of long hair	To prevent the hair becoming matted with blood

5

Post-operative complication	Altered anatomy and physiology
Haemorrhage resulting in asphyxia	The thyroid gland has an abundant blood supply and lies on either side of the trachea. Any build-up of accumulating blood from haemorrhage may cause pressure on the trachea.
Damage to recurrent laryngeal nerve resulting in respiratory obstruction	The recurrent laryngeal nerves lie in close proximity to the thyroid gland. The nerves control the laryngeal muscles opening the glottis, and voice production. Bilateral injury leads to closure of the glottis which, in turn, leads to respiratory obstruction.
Tetany	The parathyroid glands usually lie somewhere on the posterior surface of the thyroid gland. As their exact position may be unknown they are liable to damage or accidental removal. This results in hypocalcaemia which, in turn, results in increased neuromuscular irritability.
Thyroid crisis (rare)	This is attributed to a sudden release of large amounts of thyroxine into the circulation during surgery. The metabolic rate rises rapidly.

6

Observation	Significance
Blood pressure, pulse	Rapid, thready pulse and a fall in blood pressure are indicative of haemorrhage, shock and pain.
Respirations and colour	Increasing dyspnoea and respiratory rate and cyanosis may indicate laryngeal paralysis and/or compression of the trachea by accumulating blood.

Degree of restlessness and apprehension	Increasing restlessness and apprehension, if not relieved by sedation, may be a sign of impending thyroid crisis (rare).
Wound site	Fresh blood on the wound or behind the neck and shoulders is indicative of haemorrhage.
Degree of vacuum on wound drain	If the vacuum is insufficient a haematoma may form.
Hoarseness of voice	This may suggest possible nerve damage.
Evidence of tingling of toes and fingers, muscle twitching and spasms	This indicates tetany.
Fluid intake and output	A negative balance is indicative of dehydration.
First passage of urine	Urine may be retained following anaesthesia.
Temperature	A raised temperature indicates tissue damage or infection. Hyperpyrexia indicates thyroid crisis (rare).
Degree of pain	This indicates the effectiveness of analgesia.

7   Unnecessary withholding of morphine increases metabolism and restlessness and may precipitate tachycardia.
   Nursing care should be based on:
   • an individual assessment of Mrs Watson's degree and tolerance of pain
   • the likelihood of the psychological fear of moving the neck/head
   • a recognition of the factors that may increase pain, e.g. discomfort, fear of the unknown, loneliness
   Nursing actions should include:
   • moving Mrs Watson carefully
   • providing adequate support to the head when moving her
   • positioning her sitting upright with her head well supported by pillows
   • avoiding flexion of the neck

- providing a therapeutic environment which is calm, peaceful and reassuring
- providing a comfortable bed and dry, wrinkle-free bedding
- ensuring that basic needs are met, i.e. elimination, fluid and food intake, hygiene
- giving explanations and information
- spending time with Mrs Watson
- encouraging Mr Watson to visit
- teaching Mrs Watson to support her head when moving
The nurse should evaluate the care given and monitor the effects of actions and of analgesia.

8
- Give advice concerning continuation of head and neck exercises until movement is free with no pulling.
- Give advice concerning the degree of activity that can be resumed (following discussion with the surgeon). Mrs Watson should get plenty of rest in a calm, peaceful environment.
- Discuss care with Mr Watson present.
- Make an outpatient's appointment and write the date/time on a card.
Explain the importance of keeping this appointment and all future appointments.
Explain that Mrs Watson will have blood tests on all visits to test the functioning of the gland.
- Tell her about the signs of hypothyroidism, i.e. mental sluggishness, general apathy and slowness, increased sensitivity to the cold, and constipation.
- Give advice concerning when she should return to work.

Care of the Patient with Problems of the Alimentary and Biliary Tracts

3

3.1 Mr Andrews—an adult with appendicitis

Mr John Andrews, aged 32 years, has been admitted as an emergency with a suspected perforated appendix. He was taken ill at work. His wife is at home with their two young children and is unaware of his admission.

Mr Andrews is to be prepared for surgery which is to be performed as quickly as possible.

1 List the priorities of Mr Andrews' total management before he goes to theatre.
2 With reference to altered physiology explain the changes that have occurred and why Mr Andrews needs urgent surgery.
3 What is the significance of the observations carried out on Mr Andrews before surgery?
4 As part of his pre-medication Mr Andrews has been prescribed 64 mg gentamycin. The stock ampoule contains 80 mg in 2 ml. How many millilitres must be given?

Post-operatively, Mr Andrews returns from theatre following an appendicectomy. He has a nasogastric tube in situ, to be aspirated hourly, and an intravenous infusion in progress.

5 What is the relevance of Mr Andrews' post-operative observations?
6 Mr Andrews is prescribed 1 litre of dextrose/saline in 6 hours. How many drops per minute is this?
7 What are the actual and potential problems that Mr Andrews will have due to the presence of his intravenous infusion? How can such problems be cared for?
8 How can nursing care be planned to help ensure that Mr Andrews does not develop a wound infection?
9 How can the effectiveness of Mr Andrews' care be evaluated when he is ready for discharge?

3.1 Answers

1
- Relieve pain with intramuscular papaveretum 15–20 mg.
- Relieve vomiting by use of a nasogastric tube and aspiration hourly.
- Treat dehydration by intravenous infusion.
- Observe and monitor for shock and perforation.
- Prepare for theatre:
1 Gain consent and give an explanation.
2 Lock up valuables.
3 Provide a gown, and remove prosthesis and jewellery.
4 Test urine (if possible).
5 Identify the patient.

2   When the bowel is obstructed the portion proximal to the obstruction becomes distended, while the portion distal to it is empty. The portion of bowel proximal to the obstruction becomes more and more distended with accumulated digestive fluids and gas. As a result the patient's abdomen is distended. Peristalsis becomes forceful in the proximal portion to overcome the obstruction, causing severe, colicky pains. No peristalsis occurs in the distal portion, causing the patient to vomit food, gastric contents and, eventually, small bowel contents. The vomit from the small bowel is dark, thick and foul smelling because the material has been stagnant in the bowel, allowing multiplication of bacteria. The patient loses water and electrolytes through vomiting and becomes dehydrated.

Hypovolaemia and severe pain cause shock, resulting in hypotension, pallor, clamminess and a fast, thready pulse. The hypovolaemia may affect renal function and cause oliguria.

Increasing pressure on the bowel due to distension and oedema eventually impairs circulation, leading to gangrene of a portion of bowel. This necrosed bowel may perforate and the intestinal contents escape into the peritoneal cavity, causing peritonitis.

Urgent surgery is required to prevent Mr Andrews' condition from deteriorating.

3

Observation	Significance
1-hourly temperature	Mild pyrexia is usually present in appendicitis. Subnormal temperature indicates shock.

$\frac{1}{2}$-hourly pulse and blood pressure	Hypotension and tachycardia indicate deterioration due to hypovolaemia.
Colour	Increasing pallor indicates deepening shock.
1-hourly girth measurement	Increasing abdominal girth indicates peritonitis.

4   The following formula can be used:

$$\frac{\text{Dose prescribed}}{\text{Stock amount of drug}} \times \begin{array}{l}\text{number of millilitres}\\ \text{in which drug is diluted}\end{array}$$

$$= \frac{64}{80} \times 2 = \frac{64}{40}$$
$$= \frac{16}{10}$$
$$= 1.6\ \text{ml}$$

5   • **$\frac{1}{2}$-hourly respirations**   Dyspnoea and cyanosis could be a sign of asphyxia, shock or haemorrhage.
   • **$\frac{1}{2}$-hourly pulse and blood pressure**   Shock or haemorrhage may be revealed by a fast, weak pulse and low blood pressure.
   • **$\frac{1}{2}$-hourly wound check**   Excessive bleeding is indicative of reactionary haemorrhage.
   • **1-hourly aspiration of nasogastric tube**   Any blood in the aspirate may indicate internal haemorrhage.
   • **Urine output**   Observe for retention of urine.
   • **1-hourly temperature**   Slight pyrexia indicates normal reaction to surgical trauma; subnormal temperature indicates shock.
   • **Infusion**   The infusion rate should be corrected and the site observed for signs of thrombophlebitis or extravasation.

6   1 litre = 1000 ml × 15 drops (there are normally 15 drops/ml)
6 hours = 6 × 60 minutes

$$\frac{1000 \times 15}{6 \times 60} = \frac{1000}{24}$$
$$= 41.6$$
$$= \text{approximately 40 drops per minute}$$

7

Actual problem	Care
Immobility	Help with hygiene needs. Ensure that Mr Andrews' locker and belongings are in easy reach of his good side. Help with change of position every 2–4 hours. Encourage him to move his legs.
Potential problem	
Thrombophlebitis	Observe cannula site for redness, pain and swelling. Use a clean technique when handling infusion equipment.
Pulmonary oedema	Check rate is correct. Observe for dyspnoea and cough.
Extravasation	Observe cannula site for swelling or leakage of fluid. Keep site immobilized.
Cessation of flow	Keep needle site warm. Ensure that the infusion tubing is not kinked, and that the infusion bag is well above level of patient. Ask Mr Andrews not to use his limb.

8
- Do not touch original dressing for 24–48 hours.
- Plan to take dressing down when a minimum of dust is present.
- Ask patient not to touch his wound.
- Use an aseptic technique when changing dressing. Observe wound for redness, discharge and swelling.
- Observe for increasing tenderness of wound and pyrexia.

9 Mr Andrews' care can be judged as effective if the following apply when he is ready for discharge:
- There are no signs of asphyxia, haemorrhage or shock post-operatively.
- He has passed urine normally after surgery.
- His post-operative pain was well controlled.
- There have been no complications of intravenous infusion therapy.
- He was able to mobilize well from day 1 onwards.
- He was able to take diet well by day 4.
- His bowels opened on day 4 with no abdominal distension.

- He has had no dyspnoea, purulent sputum, or pyrexia.
- There has been no swelling of his calves and he has had no cause to complain of cramp.
- His wound was well healed by day 7.
- He is happy to go home on day 8. He understands that he needs 2 weeks of convalescence and that he should not lift heavy weights during this time.

3.2 Mrs Fellows—a woman with cholecystitis

Mrs Fellows, aged 45 years, has been admitted to the ward with severe abdominal colic. She has been complaining of flatulence and abdominal discomfort for some time and finds the thought and smell of fatty food often difficult to tolerate.

On examination Mrs Fellows is found to be overweight and slightly jaundiced. Her urine is dark and her stools are paler than normal. Investigations confirm the presence of gall-stones and inflammation of the gall-bladder.

1 One of the priorities of Mrs Fellows' management on admission is to relieve pain. What actions may be implemented to achieve this goal?

2 List three other problems that Mrs Fellows may have and outline the nursing actions that might be implemented.

3 With reference to altered physiology explain Mrs Fellows' presenting problems.

4 Draw a diagram to illustrate to a junior colleague the possible sites of obstruction of the biliary tract by gall-stones.

5 What advice and information should be given to Mrs Fellows on discharge regarding:
(a) her diet?
(b) the cholecystogram which is to be performed as an outpatient at a later date?

The cholecystogram confirms the presence of gall-stones and Mrs Fellows is readmitted 3 months later for a cholecystectomy and an exploration of the common bile duct.

6 How might you explain the forthcoming surgery to Mrs Fellows?

Mrs Fellows returns to the ward following surgery with an intravenous infusion in progress and a T-tube drainage system in situ.

7   One of the potential hazards of this operation is the development of hypostatic pneumonia. Explain why this is so and identify the actions that should be taken to avoid this hazard.

8   Describe, giving reasons, the role of the nurse in the care and subsequent removal of Mrs Fellows' T-tube.

9   Outline the principles of dietary management in the post-operative period and in the long term.

3.2 Answers

1
- Assess Mrs Fellows' degree of pain as measured by the systolic blood pressure, pulse, expression, colour, sweating, movement, restlessness and colic.
- Administer an analgesic, e.g. pethidine 100–150 mg i.m. every 4 hours (large doses are likely as Mrs Fellows is overweight).
- Administer anti-spasmodics, e.g. atropine, propantheline. These may be used in conjunction with an analgesic to release reflex spasm.
- Monitor the effects of the analgesia by assessing the patient as above.
- Position Mrs Fellows comfortably, with good body alignment and gentle handling.
- Allow her to discuss her worries and problems. Be available to talk and give support.
- Give adequate explanations.

2

Problem	Nursing action
Pyrexia	Well-ventilated area of ward; loose cotton clothing; extra cool fluids; fan therapy; frequent washes
Vomiting and dehydration	The withholding of all oral intake; use of a nasogastric tube; care of intravenous therapy; monitoring of fluid intake and output; administration of prescribed antiemetics.
Irritating skin due to presence of bile salts	Keeping the skin cool, clean and dry; local applications of calamine lotion; administration of antihistamines

3 The impaction of stones in the biliary system causes:
- colicky pain which radiates through to the back, under the scapula and into the right shoulder, and which is caused by spasm of the biliary ducts
- jaundice resulting from reabsorption of bile into the blood
- pruritus resulting from the accumulation of bile salts into the skin

- dark urine, where bile that has been reabsorbed into the blood is excreted via the kidney
- pale stools, where no stercobilin is available to colour the stools
- intolerance to fatty foods, and flatulence, where no bile is available for the digestion and absorption of fats

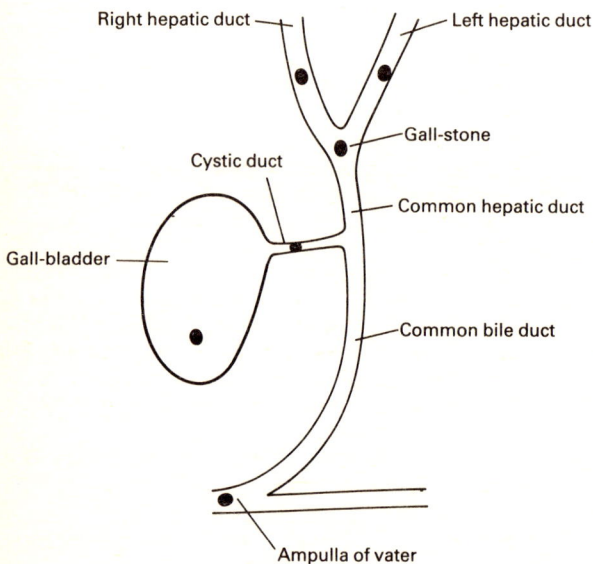

Fig. 3   The possible sites of obstruction of the biliary tract by gall-stones.

5   (a) **Diet** An appointment should be made for Mrs Fellows with the dietician and written advice should be given to her.
   Diet should be:
- low in fat as bile is not available for digestion
- low in calories. Mrs Fellows should lose weight particularly as she will probably be having surgery shortly.
- high in protein to aid and encourage wound healing
   (b) **The cholecystogram**
- Explain that the cholecystogram involves an X-ray which will show up the biliary tract. Draw a diagram to illustrate the biliary tract. Tell Mrs Fellows that this will show any gall-stones and their position in the system.

- Explain to Mrs Fellows that she will be asked to take a high fat drink just before the X rays are taken.
- Give Mrs Fellows written instructions telling her what to do the day before the test:
1 She should take the prescribed tablets (an iodine preparation, e.g. Telepaque) orally 1 hour after her evening meal which must be low in fat content. The tablets should be taken at 3–5 minute intervals with at least 250 ml of water.
2 She must have nothing to eat after her evening meal and the tablets until after the X-ray. She may drink water or black coffee.
3 If she feels nauseated, or has diarrhoea or vomiting, the test may have to be postponed.

6
- Ask Mrs Fellows what she already understands about the operation.
- Draw a simple diagram of the biliary tract.
- Explain that the operation entails removing the gall-bladder and examining the ducts for gall-stones. It is important to tell Mrs Fellows that the gall-bladder is not essential and that the only long-term implication will be that she will probably have to lower her fat intake.
- Explain the T-tube drainage system and why it will be in situ after the operation.

7   Mrs Fellows will have a tendency *not* to expand her chest fully post-operatively due to:
- obesity
- the position of incision making deep breathing painful
- reluctance to move about

This increases the likelihood of the development of hypostatic pneumonia. It is therefore advisable to take the following precautions in order to avoid this hazard:

Pre-operative care
- Discourage smoking.
- On admission, involve the physiotherapist. Teach deep breathing exercises and explain the need for coughing.

Post-operative care
- Position Mrs Fellows in such a way as to promote maximum chest expansion. Change her position from time to time.
- Administer analgesic(s) to maintain pain relief. Physiotherapy should be carried out in conjunction with analgesia.
- the physiotherapist should visit daily to encourage exercises.

- Early ambulation should be encouraged.
- Monitor Mrs Fellows for any signs of chest infection.

8 A T-tube is inserted into the common bile duct to maintain patency as the duct will be oedematous following surgery. Every day 500–700 ml of bile is produced; measuring the amount of drainage gives an indication of returning patency of the duct. After about 5 days the patency of the duct is tested by:

- clamping the tube completely, or
- raising the drainage bottle to shoulder level, or
- clamping the tube for an increasing number of hours each day.

Monitor Mrs Fellows in the following ways for indications of inadequate patency:

1 Find out if she is experiencing abdominal pain.
2 Watch the amount of drainage while unclamping the tube.
3 Test the urine for normal colour and presence of bile.
4 Observe the stools for colour.
5 Observe for the return of jaundice.

Patency of the duct is tested 6–10 days later by a T-tube cholangiogram and, if satisfactory, the tube is removed. Prepare Mrs Fellows in the following ways:

- Explain the procedure.
- Give adequate analgesia.
- Pull the tube with gentle traction. Seek advice if it is difficult to remove.

After removal, apply a dressing. Expect drainage of bile for 24–30 hours, but report it if it lasts longer. Skin may need protection with vaseline against irritating bile salts. Observe Mrs Fellows for signs of biliary peritonitis, i.e. discomfort, pain, distension.

9
- Mrs Fellows will be given only intravenous fluids initially.
- She may have a nasogastric tube in situ until bowel sounds return.
- Oral fluids are commenced about 24 hours following surgery. Begin with clear fluids and graduate to normal diet.
- While the T-tube is in situ, Mrs Fellows may have difficulty in tolerating fat, as bile is draining out and is not available for digestion, so offer her low fat food.
- Diet is discussed with the surgeon and dietician. Mrs Fellows can increase the fat content of her diet until an individual tolerance is reached.
- A reducing diet should be continued until her target weight is reached.

3.3 Antonia Benson—an adolescent with Crohn's disease

Antonia Benson, aged 16 years, has been referred to the consultant gastroenterologist for investigations of recurrent episodes of abdominal pain and diarrhoea. Antonia has been admitted to her local hospital on several occasions over the past 18 months but no diagnosis has been made. Antonia is accompanied by her parents who both work full time. She has an elder sister who is training to be a nurse and a younger brother. Antonia has just started in the sixth form at school and intends to go on to university.

On admission Antonia looks pale and thin. She weighs 48 kg compared with 54 kg a year ago. She is short for her age and complains of being listless and anorexic. Menstruation has not yet started and there is no sign of breast development.

1 Explain the significance of Antonia's social and medical history as outlined above.

2 With reference to theories of developmental psychology, identify the special needs of an adolescent such as Antonia in hospital.

3 Describe how Antonia should be prepared for colonoscopy.

Crohn's disease is confirmed following the colonoscopy. As Antonia is so underweight and unable to eat, total parenteral nutrition is commenced via a central line catheter. Antonia is prescribed prednisolone and sulphasalazine. The condition and its treatment is explained to Antonia and her parents.

4 How might Antonia react to hospitalization and the diagnosis of chronic illness, and what are the implications for nursing practice?

5 Identify the potential problems of total parenteral nutrition and, giving reasons, outline the nursing measures you would take to prevent/detect them.

6 What would be the significance of the observations you would make of Antonia during her stay in hospital in

relation to her stools, her treatment, and any potential complications.

Three weeks after admission, Antonia is ready for discharge. She is eating again and total parenteral nutrition has been discontinued. She is to be discharged home with a reducing dose of prednisolone and sulphasalazine.

7   How may the effectiveness of Antonia's care and treatment be evaluated before discharge?

8   What advice and information should Antonia be given in relation to her:
   (a)   schooling and future career?
   (b)   diet?
   (c)   treatment?

3.3 Answers

1

Information	Significance
Aged 16 years	This tells the nurse what stage of development, both physical and psychological, Antonia should have reached.
Several previous admissions with no diagnosis	Antonia will be familiar with hospitals but is likely to be depressed and maybe even frightened of tests.
Elder sister training to be a nurse; one younger brother	Antonia may well have spoken to her sister about hospital. Her sister may be able to give Antonia support. She may appreciate a visit from her brother.
Has just started sixth form; aiming for university	It is important to know what level of education Antonia has reached so that this can be continued. Antonia may be worried in case she cannot continue with her courses.
Weight 48 kg; short for age; no menstruation or breast development	Antonia should weigh about 55 kg. She is therefore well below weight. She is obviously suffering from delayed puberty and poor growth in comparison with her peers. This may well be making her depressed.

2
- **E Erikson** Proposed a series of eight psychological stages which characterizes development from the cradle to the grave. During adolescence he identifies 'finding one's identity' as the major crisis to be overcome.
- **W D Wall** Proposed the concept of the development during adolescence of the 'four selves'—the social self, sexual self, vocational self and philosophical self.
- **R G Havighurst** Lists ten developmental tasks for the adolescent period.
- **J Piaget** According to Piaget, adolescents have entered the formal concrete operational period and are capable of assuming hypothetical situations.

Needs in hospital
- Privacy

- Trusting relationships
- Independence
- Inclusion in care planning
- Contact with peer groups
- Opportunity to express feelings
- Explanations of illness and all tests
- Contact with family
- Individualized schooling and recreation

3   Explain the procedure. She will be asked to lie on her left side. Reassure her that her privacy and dignity will be maintained. She will be given some tablets before the test to sedate her. The doctor will then pass a long tube up her back passage through which he will be able to see the affected part. This may be uncomfortable but it will not be painful.

Antonia will be allowed no food for 24 hours prior to the procedure. She may drink only clear fluids. No Ribena or red-coloured drinks are allowed because they may colour the stools and mask bleeding. Antonia will be given senna syrup 24 hours before the procedure, as prescribed by the doctor.

4   Antonia's reactions may include rejection, unco-operativeness, self-assertion, withdrawal, fear, anxiety, over-confidence, depression, loneliness, boredom and aggression.

It is essential that the nurse is aware of the possible effects of hospitalization. Individualized care should be practised and time spent talking with Antonia. Her needs as described in answer 2 must be met.

5

Potential problems	Nursing actions	Rationale
Sepsis	Use a strict aseptic technique in changing dressings and in connection of new giving sets, which should be renewed every 24 to 48 hours. 4-hourly temperature recordings.	To reduce the risk of infection

Hyperglycaemia	Make frequent blood sugar estimations and urinalysis.	To monitor for signs of hyperglycaemia
Rupture of pleural membrane following insertion of cannula	Report any cyanosis, breathlessness or pain immediately.	To determine the degree of pneumothorax
Air embolism	Ensure that no air gets into the system when changing it. This prevents disconnections in the line.	To prevent air from entering the system
Overinfusion of fluids	Maintain a strict intake chart; regulate the rate of infusion as prescribed; use an infusion pump; weigh Antonia daily.	To prevent fluid from being infused too rapidly and to monitor any signs of overhydration

6

Observation	Significance
Stools	Stools that increase in frequency and loose stools containing blood/mucus indicate ineffectiveness of therapy. Blood in the stools may indicate haemorrhage. Cessation of bowel movements may indicate intestinal obstruction.
Pulse	Tachycardia may indicate perforation or generalized peritonitis.
Blood pressure	Hypertension may be a side-effect of steroids.

Urinalysis	Glycosuria is a side-effect of steroids.
Leakage of faecal fluid via the vagina or urethra	This is indicative of fistula formation.

7   The following criteria should be considered:
   - Antonia's ability to tolerate oral food
   - Any weight gain
   - Whether there is a reduced number of stools which are better formed. No blood or mucus should be present.
   - The extent to which Antonia is able to look after her own treatment and understand the importance of continued treatment
   - The extent to which she is able to discuss her feelings and anxieties
   - Whether there have been any complications of total parenteral nutrition

8   (a)   There is no reason why Antonia should not continue with her exams and with her future plans for university. She may require periods in hospital during which her education will be continued.

   (b)   Antonia should see the dietician before discharge to discuss her diet. She may require supplements, e.g. iron, vitamin B_{12}, folic acid and fat-soluble vitamins. She may take a normal diet but she should omit any food known to exacerbate the disease. She may require a high protein/high carbohydrate diet while she is underweight.

   (c)   Antonia must continue to take the steroids as prescribed and must carry a card with the details of her treatment on it. She must not stop taking them at any time unless instructed to do so by the doctor.

   If she feels ill she should go to see her doctor as he may have to increase her dose of steroids.

   She should take her tablets with food.

   Antonia should be warned about a probable generalized weight gain and a 'moon face', which will decrease with reduced treatment.

3.4 Mrs Rogers—an adult with diverticulitis

Mrs Ethel Rogers, aged 62 years, is admitted to the ward as an emergency with acute abdominal pain. Acute diverticulitis is diagnosed.

Mrs Rogers is a widow who lives at home with her elderly father who needs almost constant supervision. On admission she is anxious, in severe constant pain, and has a temperature of 38.5°C. An intravenous infusion is commenced and a nasogastric tube is passed. Mrs Rogers is to have nothing to eat or drink. Pethidine is prescribed for pain.

1   What actions should the nurse take to ensure that Mrs Rogers' father is looked after during her stay in hospital?
2   With reference to research what methods might be used to evaluate Mrs Rogers' pain and the effectiveness of the pethidine?
3   Discuss how Mrs Rogers should be prepared for the passage of the nasogastric tube and be encouraged to cooperate.
4   Describe the specific care Mrs Rogers will require with regard to the nasogastric tube.
5   List the nursing actions that might be implemented to reduce Mrs Rogers' temperature.

Four days after admission, Mrs Rogers starts eating again, the intravenous infusion is discontinued, and the nasogastric tube is removed. A high fibre diet is prescribed.

6   With reference to altered anatomy and physiology explain why a low fibre diet is contraindicated.
7   Outline a dietary plan for Mrs Rogers to follow when she gets home.

While in hospital Mrs Rogers confides that she is finding it increasingly difficult to look after her father. She explains that he is incontinent and that she is unable to lift him into the bath.

8   How might Mrs Rogers be helped to care for her father at home?

9   How might you explain Mrs Rogers' condition, its treatment and its potential complications to the junior nurse who has been assigned to work with you?

3.4 Answers

1 • Find out if Mrs Rogers has any other relatives who could look after her father. Ask her if there is anybody else who could care for him.
 • Contact the social worker and give her details about Mrs Rogers' father.
 • Ensure that her father is aware of what is happening to his daughter.
 • Arrange for him to visit Mrs Rogers.

2 'Pain is what the patient says it is and exists when he says it does' (McCaffery, 1983). Pain is subjective and assessment is required to find out an individual's response to pain. Pain should be assessed *with* the patient; his verbal report of his own pain is the most reliable indicator (Jacox, 1979).

 The effectiveness of the pethidine must be assessed so that it can be administered according to Mrs Rogers' individual needs.

 Methods of assessing pain are as follows:
 • pain assessment chart
 • pain description chart
 • visual, analogue scale (Scott and Huskisson, 1976)
 • pain profile (Bond, 1979)
 • pain relief description (Loan and Dundee, 1967)

3 **Assess**
 • Talk to Mrs Rogers about her worries and fears.
 • Ask her about previous experiences.
 • Ask if she is allergic to strapping.

 Plan
 • Explain the purpose of the tube and what to expect during and after insertion of the tube, and explain that the tube will be passed via her nostril.
 • Explain that she will still be able to clean her teeth.

 Implement
 • Explain that insertion will be easier if she relaxes, breathes deeply via her mouth, and swallows when instructed.
 • Tell her that sips of water may help her to swallow.
 Allow Mrs Rogers to ask questions before you commence.

4 • Ensure that the tube is secured to Mrs Rogers' face so as to be comfortable. Use hypo-allergenic tape and watch the skin carefully for any signs of irritation.
 • Ensure that there is no tension or pulling on the tube, especially when Mrs Rogers moves around in bed.

- Encourage normal teeth cleaning and 2-hourly mouth-washes (more frequently if required).
- Apply petroleum jelly or glycerine to Mrs Rogers' lips to prevent them from becoming dry and sore.
- Cleanse Mrs Rogers' nostril gently with normal saline or water.
- Encourage Mrs Rogers to change her position in bed. This relieves pressure on one area of the throat.
- Monitor the amount of drainage from the tube and aspirate the tube as directed. Note the characteristics of the aspirate.

5
- Turn down any radiators near her bed.
- Ensure that she wears light, cotton nightclothes.
- Reduce the number of sheets/blankets on the bed.
- Open a nearby window provided there are no draughts.
- Offer her ice to suck.
- Give her frequent cool washes.
- Use a fan to cool circulating air. (If Mrs Rogers shivers, turn off the fan.)

6   A fibre-deficient diet results in small, hard stools which take a long time to pass through the large bowel and are voided with effort. High intracolonic pressures are therefore needed in order to expel these faeces. A long period of time of being subjected to these pressures leads to herniation of the mucosa and the development of pouches and diverticula. Fibre in the diet forms cellulose which absorbs water. This swells and softens the stools which makes them easier to pass, and stimulates peristalsis.

7   Mrs Rogers should be given written advice on the high fibre diet. There is no reason why her father could not eat the same food, so there is no need to cook different meals for him. The following dietary advice should be given:
- 100% wholemeal bread and bran-containing cereals, e.g. All Bran, should be included in the diet.
- Bran can be added to their food, beginning with 2 tea-spoonfuls three times a day. This should be increased until they defecate twice a day without straining.
- Bran can be prescribed in tablet form which should be chewed and washed down with fluids. These will be useful for Mrs Rogers if she is away from home.
- She should eat plenty of fruit and vegetables but should avoid sugar and refined flour.
- Mrs Rogers should be encouraged to eat foods high in fibre, e.g. baked potatoes, parsnips, peas, beans and pulses.

8 Members of the primary health care team must be informed of Mrs Rogers' difficulties. The following services are available to help her:
  ● laundry service
  ● home help
  ● district nurse to assist with lifting her father into the bath
  ● social worker to help Mrs Rogers get aid, e.g. a hoist, and to ensure that Mrs Rogers gets her full attendance allowances
  ● day-care facilities for Mrs Rogers' father to enable her to have some time to herself
  ● self-help groups for people with similar problems
9 Find out what the nurse already knows by asking her questions.
  ● Provide explanations either while caring for Mrs Rogers or in a more formal situation in a quiet area of the ward.
  ● Explain the condition, perhaps by using a diagram similar to Fig. 4.

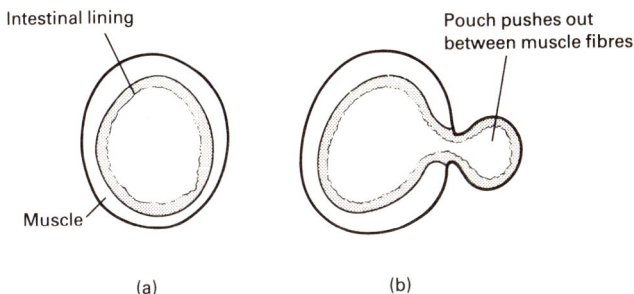

Fig. 4 (a) Cross section through a normal bowel. (b) Cross section through a bowel with a diverticulum (pouch).

Explain that the condition is caused by a fibre-deficient diet, which makes stools hard. Intracolonic pressure is increased to expel the faeces and this leads to the formation of diverticula. The diverticula have become inflamed, causing the clinical features of an acute abdominal problem.
  ● The following forms of treatment can then be discussed:
  1 conservative management with diet alone
  2 rest, antibiotics, gastric suction and intravenous therapy if obstructed
  3 surgery, which may be performed at a later date when the acute phase has passed
  4 the prescription of a high fibre diet

- The nurse should then be given some reading and the effectiveness of teaching should be evaluated by asking questions and/or giving a quiz.
- The complications that should be pointed out to the nurse include:
  1 pericolic abscess
  2 purulent pericolitis
  3 perforation leading to faecal peritonitis/haemorrhage
  4 fistulas between colon and the bladder, vagina or renal tract

3.5 Mr Wells—a man with a duodenal ulcer

Mr Graham Wells, aged 42 years, is a sheet metal worker in a local factory. The factory is making men redundant and Mr Wells has been worrying about his job for some months now. Mr Wells is married with two young children and his wife is expecting their third child in 2 months time. Mr Wells was diagnosed as having a duodenal ulcer about 2 years ago and since then his health has been fairly good. However, since his worries have increased, he has started smoking again and is drinking more than usual. He was admitted 2 weeks ago, having collapsed at home following the passage of a large melaena. A blood transfusion was given and the bleeding ceased. He has now been readmitted following a further episode of melaena.

On admission, Mr Wells is obviously severely shocked. His pulse is 110 beats/min and his blood pressure is 80/60 mmHg. He is anxious, frightened and a little confused as to his whereabouts. Mr Wells is to be prepared for surgery as soon as his condition allows it. A blood transfusion is commenced.

1 List the specific information the nurse would need to gain from Mr Wells on admission.
2 What nursing actions would be taken to reduce Mr Wells' anxiety levels pre-operatively?
3 Giving reasons, select four essential items from the following possible nursing actions to indicate how Mr Wells should be prepared for emergency surgery:
   - Perform a pubic shave.
   - Weigh him.
   - Take baseline observations.
   - Give him a bed bath.
   - Check that the consent form has been signed.
   - Administer an enema.
   - Administer the pre-medication.
   - Test his urine.
   - Identify him.
   - Remove false teeth and jewellery.
   - Pass a nasogastric tube.
   - Teach deep breathing exercises.
4 With reference to altered physiology explain how Mr Wells' body has responded to the melaena.

Mr Wells is taken to theatre 1½ hours after admission, where an antrectomy is performed.

5 Identify the actions that will be taken in theatre in order to ensure Mr Wells' safety and comfort.

Mr Wells returns to the ward with a nasogastric tube and intravenous infusion in situ. His wife is waiting at his bedside and is obviously distressed.

6 Discuss how Mrs Wells can be reassured about her husband's condition and how her needs may be met.

7 Describe, giving reasons, how Mr Wells might be mobilized post-operatively.

Mr Wells makes an uneventful recovery and is ready for discharge 2 weeks after admission.

8 What advice and information should Mr Wells be given on discharge?

9 What support is available in the community for Mr Wells and his family should he be made redundant?

3.5 Answers

1   • His name, age, address and home telephone number for contacting relatives
     • Whether or not he has had surgery before
     • Any allergies of which he is aware
     • When he last ate or drank and what it was
     • Whether his wife is with him/whether she knows about his admission

2   • Explain exactly what has happened to him and what is to happen. Explain all procedures.
     • Administer prescribed sedation to alleviate pain and apprehension. Ensure that he is comfortable.
     • Contact his wife/encourage her to sit with him.
     • Ensure that somebody is looking after the children.
     • Inform the factory.

3   • Identify him—to ensure that he is given the correct treatment.
     • Remove any false teeth—to prevent any obstruction to his airway during and after anaesthesia.
     • Remove any jewellery—to reduce the risk of loss and electric burns from the diathermy machine.
     • Check that the consent form has been signed (although it is not the nurse's responsibility to get the consent form signed).
     • Administer pre-medication—to allay anxiety.

4   Loss of blood from the circulating volume stimulates:
     • the sympathetic nervous system and the release of adrenaline and noradrenaline from the adrenal medulla
     • the release of renin which converts angiotensinogen into angiotensin
       These in turn cause:
     • widespread selective vasoconstriction in vessels in the skin, lungs, gastrointestinal tract, liver and kidneys, leading to pale skin, reduced peristalsis, and oliguria
     • selective vasoconstriction ensuring a greater volume of blood to the heart and brain
     • stimulated sweat glands, resulting in clammy skin
     • an increase in the rate and force of contraction of the heart, leading to tachycardia. A reduction in blood pressure stimulates the production of antidiuretic hormone from the posterior lobe of the pituitary gland and aldosterone from the adrenal gland, which increases the reabsorption of sodium and water to conserve body fluid.

- anaerobic metabolism in the tissues, leading to the accumulation of harmful metabolites, i.e. metabolic acidosis
- a reduction of blood pressure, leading to oliguria or anuria

5
- Safety, comfort and privacy should be ensured on the theatre trolley.
- Mr Wells should never be left alone at any time.
- Correct identification must be ensured.
- The nurse must be aware of the toxic effects of anaesthesia.
- Static electricity should be prevented.
- Mr Wells must be kept warm.
- He must be positioned correctly and carefully on the table.
- Asepsis must be maintained.
- Swabs and equipment must be correctly counted.
- A clear airway must be maintained following surgery.
- Mr Wells should be reassured while he is regaining consciousness.
- Any injury from thrashing of limbs during recovery should be prevented.
- Full instructions must be given to the collecting nurse.

6
- Encourage Mrs Wells to stay at her husband's bedside.
- Explain the infusion, the nasogastric tube and the position of his wound.
- Explain all that you do for him to avoid her becoming anxious.
- Assure her that he will be kept free from pain.
- Explain briefly what has been done, and ask the surgeon to talk to her to tell her the result of the surgery. Stay with her during this talk to be available to answer questions.
- Provide her with a comfortable chair and the chance to put her feet up and relax.
- Offer her a cup of tea. Make sure she has her meals and that she knows where the toilets are.

7   Activity and frequent changes of position should be promoted, as should early ambulation to reduce predisposition to:
- retention of urine
- abdominal distension
- loss of strength
- joint stiffness
- respiratory and vascular complications
- sluggish peristalsis

- venous stasis.

In the early post-operative period Mr Wells should be encouraged to sit up when fully conscious and when his blood pressure is satisfactory. This aids lung expansion and reduces the possibility of chest infections.

Foot and leg exercises should be encouraged to prevent deep vein thrombosis. Mr Wells may be assisted out of bed after 24–48 hours depending on his condition. Movement is increased as he feels more able. Adequate pain relief must be given. He should not be left alone during the early stages of mobilization in case he feels dizzy and falls.

8
- Mr Wells should avoid eating fibrous foods, (e.g. citrus fruits, skins and seeds) as they cannot be digested by gastric tissue.
- He should chew his food properly to aid digestion.
- He should be given information about 'dumping syndrome' and the following advice as to what to do about it:
1 Eat small, frequent meals and avoid meals that are high in sugars and salts.
2 Reduce the amount of fluids taken with meals but take them between meals.
3 Eat slowly and rest after meals.
4 Take any drugs prescribed to reduce gastric motility.
- It should be explained to Mr Wells that he will get drunk more quickly with alcohol.
- He should be advised to keep his follow-up appointments.
- He should be told to see his general practitioner if he has any problems.

9 Supplementary benefit, which will also entitle the family to:
1 help towards housing costs
2 extra help towards heating costs
3 free NHS dental treatment
4 free prescriptions
5 free school meals
6 lump sums to help with clothes for the new baby
- Unemployment benefit
- Redundancy payment

3.6 Mrs Armitage—a woman with haemorrhoids

Mrs Armitage, aged 52 years, has been admitted to the ward for haemorrhoidectomy. She has only fairly recently attended her general practitioner and has been suffering from pain, itching and bleeding for several years.

She is married with three grown-up children and has a part-time job. On admission, Mrs Armitage is noted to have a considerable amount of money with her and several pieces of jewellery. She is also extremely anxious about the forthcoming surgery.

1 With reference to your responsibilities what actions would you take in relation to Mrs Armitage's valuables?
2 What actions might be taken to allay Mrs Armitage's anxiety pre-operatively?
3 Describe the nurse's role during a rectal examination and proctoscopy which is performed after admission.

During Mrs Armitage's stay, you are asked to give a tutorial to a group of four nurses, all of whom are at different stages of training.

4 With reference to the principles of learning how would you plan and carry out this teaching session?
5 With reference to altered physiology what would you tell them about the predisposing factors of haemorrhoids?

Mrs Armitage returns from theatre following surgical excision of haemorrhoids.

6 Identifying the problems (actual/potential) draw up a care plan to show the specific care that Mrs Armstrong will require post-operatively.

7 What discharge arrangements should you make when Mrs Armitage is ready to go home 4 days later?

3.6   Answers

1   Neither the nurse nor the hospital has any legal responsibilities towards Mrs Armitage's valuables and neither is liable should anything go missing. The patient is responsible for any items which he/she brings into the hospital. However, it is reasonable for the nurse to take precautions to protect patients' belongings.

This situation should be explained to Mrs Armitage so that she understands the implications. She should be encouraged to ask her husband to take home all the jewellery and most of the money to ensure their safe-keeping. If she is not able to do this then all her valuables should be catalogued by two nurses and locked away in a ward safe/special drawer.

2   ● Talk to Mrs Armitage and find out what she knows and understands about the operation. Straighten out any misconceptions and explain the operation again.
● Involve Mrs Armitage in her pre-operative preparation, with explanations of all procedures.
● Involve Mr Armitage in discussions so that he may support his wife.
● Explain what to expect after the operation and explain that pain will be controlled. She may be very worried about having her bowels open post-operatively.
● Administer night sedation as prescribed. Take actions to ensure a good night's rest.

3   A rectal examination will be uncomfortable and undignified for Mrs Armitage so the nurse must take this into consideration. Privacy must be ensured with no chance of interruption. The procedure and its purpose must be explained to Mrs Armitage. She should be instructed to lie on her left side in a curled position with the inner surface of the right knee resting on the couch. She should be covered apart from the buttocks. Dignity must be maintained at all times. The nurse should talk to Mrs Armitage during the procedure to reassure her and keep her informed of what the doctor is doing.

4

Principle	Planning and implementation
Students must be motivated to learn	Give the students incentive by indicating: 1 what they will know after the session 2 the relevance of the material

Basic needs must be met before learning will take place.	Ensure a warm room, somewhere to sit, that the nurses are not hungry/thirsty, and that it is not the end of the day.
Students learn by being active.	Plan to involve the students and encourage participation, e.g. in the form of question/answer sessions.
Students must be attending to what you are teaching.	Ensure a quiet area of the ward. Choose a time of day when students are not busy or preoccupied with other work.
Perception is important.	Ensure that the students can see what you are doing and that they follow you. Make use of the senses in teaching.
The session must be structured so that it is easier to remember.	Plan the session in logical steps, building upon previous knowledge. Summarize the information at the end.
Students need to practise.	Plan time for them to consolidate work and to do extra reading etc. Provide reading references.
Students need feedback as to their progress.	Use questions and answers at the end of the session to recap. Set extra work and test them on it.

5   The haemorrhoidal veins act as collateral connections between the portal and systemic venous systems. The portal venous system has no valves; therefore, increased intra-abdominal pressure is transmitted directly to these veins by gravity.

Increased pressure causes distension of the veins. Continuous pressure causes varicosities.

The predisposing factors that cause increased intra-abdominal pressure and can therefore lead to haemorrhoids are:

- straining to defecate, i.e. constipation
- coughing/sneezing
- obesity
- pregnancy
- portal hypertension

- tumours in the abdominal cavity
- straining to micturate
- heavy lifting work
- prolonged standing, resulting in raised rectal venous pressure due to gravity

6

Problem (actual/potential)	Nursing action
Pain and discomfort	Administer analgesia as prescribed and at the specified times. Move Mrs Armitage gently. Encourage warm hip-baths after 24 hours. Move from side to side. Use sheepskin.
Potential haemorrhage	Observe dressings for signs of haemorrhage. Monitor vital signs to detect any haemorrhage as soon as possible. Take pulse hourly and blood pressure as directed.
Potential infection	Mrs Armitage should take a warm bath after all bowel motions and a fresh pad should be applied. Monitor her temperature.
Fear of pain on defecation	Encourage bowel activity by encouraging food as soon as possible (including fruit and fluids). Administer aperients as prescribed. These actions will promote a soft stool which will be easier to pass. Analgesia should be continued until defecation has been achieved.
Possible retention of urine	Encourage Mrs Armitage to get out of bed to go to the toilet. Warm baths may help. Ensure privacy.
Possible stricture formation	Mrs Armitage may be taught how to use an anal dilator.

7
- Educate of Mrs Armitage before discharge regarding:
1 perianal hygiene
2 diet to prevent constipation
3 adequate fluid intake and exercise
- Discuss aftercare with Mr and Mrs Armitage.

- Communicate an agreed plan of aftercare with the community contact.
- Arrange an outpatient appointment and give Mrs Armitage the date and time of this appointment.
- Arrange for the supply of any drugs to be taken home.
- Arrange transport if necessary.
- Give Mrs Armitage a date and time for discharge from hospital.

3.7   Mr Church—a man with a strangulated hernia

Mr Church, aged 58 years, is a porter at a large local airport. He has been on the waiting list to have surgery for an inguinal hernia for 18 months. However, over the past 2 days he has been increasingly unwell. He has been vomiting and has had severe abdominal pain with abdominal distension and no bowel movements.

On admission Mr Church is frightened, anxious, pale and sweating. His blood pressure is 100/70 mmHg and his pulse is 100 beats/min and thready. He is vomiting green-brown fluid and his urine is dark and concentrated. His mouth is dry and he complains of thirst. He has been accompanied to the ward by his wife.

1   Explain how a junior colleague could be helped to prepare for Mr Church's admission into the ward.
2   What explanation could you give to Mrs Church if she asks what has happened and why her husband needs urgent surgery?
3   Explain the significance of the information given above which was gained during an initial nursing assessment.
4   Outline, giving reasons, the essential pre-operative nursing actions that will be implemented when preparing Mr Church for surgery.

Mr Church goes to theatre 4 hours after admission, where the hernia is reduced and a resection of bowel is performed. He has an intravenous infusion of whole blood in progress and the nasogastric tube is on free drainage.

5   List the nurse's responsibilities when collecting Mr Church from theatre.
6   Identify, giving reasons, the nursing actions that may be implemented to reduce/prevent the possible effects of immobilization following surgery.

Eight days following surgery Mr Church suddenly complains of 'something giving way' and a warm feeling on his skin. On examination you find that his wound has burst open at one end and a small portion of bowel has eviscerated.

7 List the factors that may have predisposed to wound dehiscence.

8 What actions should the nurse take in this situation?

Mr Church returns to theatre, where the wound is resutured with the addition of deep tension sutures. Following this he makes a good recovery.

9 What advice and information should Mr Church be given when he is fully recovered and ready for home?

3.7   Answers

1 • Ask your colleague what she already knows about
     strangulated hernias and the condition in which she
     expects to find Mr Church on arrival in the ward. Expand
     on her knowledge as necessary.
   • Identify the potential problems Mr Church may have.
   • Prepare a bed area near the nurses' station.
   • Ask the student to collect together all necessary equip-
     ment and charts.
   • Check that all essential items are available.
   • Help her to assess Mr Church's priorities on admission.
   • Allow her to ask questions throughout.
   • Assess her learning by either arranging a mock situation
     or by watching her prepare for another similar admission.
   • Direct her to relevant reading, e.g. books, articles.

2 Firstly find out what Mrs Church already knows about an
   inguinal hernia. It may then be useful to draw a diagram
   of a hernia to show protrusion of bowel through a weakness
   in the wall of the abdomen. Explain that a hernia often
   arises as a result of chronic coughing or heavy lifting, which
   increases the pressure within the abdominal cavity.

   Once Mrs Church understands the concept of a hernia
   you can then go on to explain strangulation. Tell her that
   the neck of the hernial sac has become constricted (use a
   diagram or model), thereby causing an obstruction of the
   bowel. The blood supply to this portion of bowel has been
   interrupted. Because the bowel has become obstructed,
   nothing can pass through it; hence the vomiting and no
   bowel movement. It is therefore vital to operate to remove
   the obstruction.

3

Information	Significance
He is a porter at an airport.	He probably has to lift heavy objects, and this is likely to have been a predisposing factor in the development of his hernia. He will have to avoid heavy lifting when he eventually returns to work.
He has been on the waiting list for surgery.	He will know about his inguinal hernia; this will make explanations easier.

He has been vomiting and has had severe abdominal pain with distension and no bowel movements.	These are all indicative of intestinal obstruction caused by a strangulated hernia.
He is pale and sweating, his BP is 100/70 mmHg, and his pulse is 100 beats/min and thready.	These are all indicative of shock caused by pain and dehydration.
He has been vomiting green-brown fluid.	This is indicative of intestinal obstruction.
His urine is dark and concentrated, and he has a dry mouth and thirst.	These are indicative of dehydration.
He has been accompanied by his wife.	She will be anxious and will need to be involved in his care. She will also need explanations and reassurance.

4

Nursing action	Rationale
Ensure that Mr Church is wearing an identification bracelet with correct information.	To prevent misidentification, which could lead to possible harm
Assist Mr Church into a theatre gown (cotton).	To reduce the risk of infection and to ensure that he is not wearing any nylon.
Remove any false teeth.	To prevent trauma during anaesthesia.
Remove any jewellery.	To prevent accidental loss of jewellery, and trauma to the patient, e.g. diathermy burns
Test urine if possible for glucose and protein	To detect diabetes (indicated by glucose in the urine) and to detect renal disease (indicated by protein in the urine)

Check that he has signed a consent form.	To comply with legal requirements
Administer pre-medication as prescribed.	To allay anxiety and reduce oral secretions

5
- Ascertain exactly which operation has been done.
- Ask for instructions regarding immediate care of the intravenous infusion and nasogastric tube.
- Ascertain the number and type of wound drains in situ. Observe the wound.
- Ask if any analgesia has been administered. If so, what and when?
- Collect notes/operation information (according to hospital policy).
- Check Mr Church's condition, i.e. pulse, colour, respirations.
- Ensure that Mr Church's airway is patent before leaving the recovery area.
  If unhappy with his condition do not take him back to the ward.
- Ensure safety and comfort and a clear airway on his return journey to the ward.

6

Possible effects	Nursing action	Rationale
Stasis of respiratory secretions leading to infection	Assist to a sitting position during the first 12 hours post-operatively.	This aids lung expansion.
	Supporting the wound, encourage deep breathing and coughing 2-hourly.	This aids full lung expansion and the removal of secretions.
Venous stasis, particularly in the lower limbs.	Encourage foot and leg exercises after 12 hours. Mr Church should continue these 2-hourly until he is mobile.	This stimulates circulation and venous return.

| | Prevent excess weight on the lower limbs and discourage him from crossing his legs in bed. | This prevents obstruction to venous return. |
| Pressure sores | Turn Mr Church from side to side 2-hourly; encourage him to lift his bottom off the bed; keep the sheets wrinkle free; use sheepskins; keep his skin clean. | All these actions reduce the possibility of prolonged pressure in one area. |

7 • Wound infection
   • Age of patient
   • Post-operative vomiting
   • Post-operative ileus
   • Coughing
   • Straining at defecation
   • Suturing technique

8 • Reassure Mr Church and explain to him what has happened. Someone should remain with him.
   • Inform the surgeon.
   • Cover the wound with sterile dressings soaked in normal saline.
   • Ask Mr Church to lie still.
   • Tell the surgeon when Mr Church last ate or drank.
   • Prepare Mr Church for surgery and resuturing of the wound.
   • Inform his wife of the situation.

9 Mr Church should not return to work for at least 1 month and after he has had a check-up in the outpatient department.
   • He should be discouraged from lifting heavy objects. If this is going to be difficult when back at work, he should be taught good lifting techniques.

- If he is a smoker, he should be encouraged to give up or at least cut down on cigarettes.
- He must be given an outpatient's appointment date.
- All information should be written down, as well as given verbally.

4 Care of the Patient with a Mental or Physical Handicap

4.1   Martin Newsome—a young man with cerebral palsy

Martin Newsome, aged 19 years, has cerebral palsy. He was diagnosed as having spastic quadraplegia when he was 5 months old and has been cared for by his parents ever since. He has two younger sisters aged 10 and 14 years. Martin has been admitted to the ward for 2 weeks while his family go on holiday. This is the first time that the family have had a holiday, leaving Martin in hospital, and Mrs Newsome is extremely anxious about him and says she feels guilty.

Martin has an IQ of 80 but is severely retarded physically. He is toilet trained but is unable to use a bottle or the toilet on his own. He is unable to walk and spends much of his time in his special chair. He is also unable to feed himself, but lately has shown an eagerness to try. Communication with Martin is difficult as he is not able to speak.

1   What response would you make to Mrs Newsome when she admits to feeling anxious and guilty about leaving Martin?

2   What information must the nurse find out from Mr and Mrs Newsome before they leave, in order to meet Martin's needs for the next 2 weeks?

3   With reference to altered physiology how would you explain Martin's condition to the junior nurses on the ward?

4   What would Mr and Mrs Newsome have been told about the causes of cerebral palsy and the risk to future children before they had their second child?

Exercise and correct positioning are extremely important to consider when planning Martin's care.

5   How should Martin be positioned when he is:
   (a)   sitting in his chair?
   (b)   lying down?

6   Outline the principles involved in feeding Martin and the ways in which he can be encouraged to become more independent in this activity of living.

7 List the methods available to help an individual with cerebral palsy to overcome communication difficulties.

8 What may have been the effects on the family of coping with Martin, and how may they have been helped to cope?

When Mr and Mrs Newsome arrive to collect Martin, he is obviously pleased to see them.

---

9 What information should be passed on to Martin's parents before they take him home?

4.1   Answers

1   It is very important that the family do not feel guilty about leaving Martin. Emphasize that it is essential that they have a break from caring for Martin and that they relax. Ensure them that Martin will be well cared for. Explain that they will be able to care for him more easily if they have had a good rest. A stay in hospital will give the hospital team a chance to reassess Martin and help with any problems. It will also give Martin a chance to meet new people and other children. The staff could also try to develop Martin's feeding ability. Suggest that Mrs Newsome leaves something personal with Martin as tangible evidence of her continued love and as evidence that she will return.

2

Need	Information required
Eating and drinking	What sort of food does he have? Can he chew? How has he shown eagerness to help himself? What food/drinks does he like/dislike? At what time of the day does he have his meals? What is the best way to feed him?
Elimination	How does he indicate the need to use a bottle/the toilet? What is the best way to get him on/off the toilet? How often does he usually have his bowels opened? Does he suffer from constipation?
Communication	How does he communicate his needs? Has he any special words/non-verbal behaviour? Has he any other methods of communicating, e.g. picture cards?
Hygiene and dressing	How does Mrs Newsome normally manage with him in the bath? How often does he have a bath/his hair washed/his teeth cleaned? Does he like his bath? What sort of clothes are easiest for him to wear? How much does he do for himself?
Play/education	What level of development is he at? What are his favourite games/toys? What education does he normally have?

Sleep and rest	What time does he go to bed? How long does he sleep for? In what position does he sleep most soundly? Are there any particular problems? Does he take any medication?
Safety	How capable is he of protecting himself from dangers? Does he have cot sides to his bed? What understanding of safety does he have?
Mobility	What is the best way to move/lift him? What exercises does he have? How is he best positioned? Does he have calipers? Is he able to walk at all?

3 Cerebral palsy is a motor function disorder caused by damage to the immature brain before, during, or shortly after birth. The effects on the individual will depend on the area of brain damaged. In Martin's case the effect is spasticity affecting all four limbs. The area of the brain damaged is the corticol motor area and/or the pyramidal tract (draw a diagram to show these areas), causing abnormally strong tone of certain muscle groups. Any attempt to move a joint causes the muscles to contract, and the movement is blocked. It is important to stress that Martin is not paralysed. His IQ indicates that he is mildly retarded.

4 It is impossible to guarantee that subsequent children will not be affected by cerebral palsy. Having had Martin, however, does not make Mrs Newsome any more likely to have a second affected child—cerebral palsy is not inherited. Mr and Mrs Newsome will have been told the causes of cerebral palsy, which can be divided into three main categories:

1 **Pre-natal causes**, e.g. maternal infection due to viral or infectious agents, metabolic disease

2 **Natal causes**, e.g. anoxia due to cord around the neck, asphyxia, trauma during delivery, prematurity

3 **Post-natal causes**, e.g. trauma, childhood infections

Once the parents had had a chance to ask questions they would have had to make up their own minds about future children.

5 (a) Martin should be placed well back in his chair and thigh straps utilized if he has difficulty staying there. The pelvis should be held symmetrically with the weight taken evenly

by both ischial tuberosities. His head should be supported if necessary in an upright position and in the midline. Martin should not spend all day in his chair; instead, opportunities should be taken to place him in other positions.

(b) It is important to find out the most suitable position for Martin when he is lying down. Again, different positions should be tried and Martin encouraged to move. Laying Martin on his stomach will enable him to try to lift his head to look around, and it will be easier for him to straighten his hips and legs. There will be less tendency for the legs to assume the closed position. He should not ideally be laid on his back. The preferred position is between the lateral and supine position. He will need to be moved regularly depending on his ability to move on his own.

6   Martin should be placed in a suitable position, sitting upright with his head in the midline. The nurse should sit directly in front of Martin to encourage maintenance of the midline position. All food and utensils should also be placed directly in front of him. Advice should be followed from parents regarding the diet and method of feeding. Food should not be too hot or too cold. Foods with a high sugar content should be avoided as this increases salivation. Appropriate utensils should be used, e.g. Teflon-coated spoons, cut-out cups (allow feeder to empty the cup by tilting the cup rather than the head).

To encourage Martin to feed himself, he should be given finger foods and utensils with large handles to improve the grip. Foods should be thick enough to stay on the spoon. The nurse should assist Martin with guiding the food to his mouth, give him plenty of time and encouragement, and not show impatience.

7   • Blissymbolics (a picture and idea system which can be used on communication boards or electronic displays)
    • Simple picture cards/flash cards
    • Speech synthesizers
    • Typewriters
    • Involvement of speech therapists

8   • Tiredness
    • Social isolation both for parents and siblings
    • Failure to meet their own needs—life revolves around Martin.
    • Feelings of neglect and jealousy from siblings. They may have difficulty at school and show aggression or difficult behaviour.
    • Marital problems. This may have pushed Mr and Mrs

Newsome apart. On the other hand, it may have drawn them closer together.
- Financial difficulties.

Help and support may have included:
- help from social services regarding finance, aids and appliances, and housing
- help from charitable funds
- support from physiotherapists and occupational therapists
- home sitting service, voluntary agencies, and self-help groups
- community nursing services
- societies for the handicapped

9
- Information about how he has been and any problems that may have arisen
- Information regarding any progress made with feeding
- Information regarding any assessment and its results
- Any changes in possible medication

4.2   Mrs Stuart—an elderly lady who has had a cerebrovascular accident

Mrs Ethel Stuart, aged 72 years, lives with her husband in a small terraced house about 15 miles from the hospital. They have no children and no close relatives living nearby.

Mrs Stuart has had mitral stenosis for the past 10 years, and apart from becoming breathless after exertion on a few occasions, she has been perfectly well until now. She has been admitted to the ward accompanied by her husband after he found her collapsed at home.

On admission, she is drowsy, slightly confused, dysphasic and has a dense right-sided hemiplegia. Mr Stuart, aged 81 years, is extremely anxious about his wife and reluctant to leave her.

1   What information should be elicited during the initial nursing assessment of Mrs Stuart?
2   What nursing actions might be implemented to overcome Mrs Stuart's problem of communication on admission?
3   List four of the important nursing problems Mrs Stuart may have on admission.
4   With reference to altered physiology explain the reasons for these problems.
5   Mr Stuart asks what will happen to his wife. How can you best answer him?

Forty-eight hours later Mrs Stuart is fully conscious and alert. She still has difficulty in communicating and moving her right side.

6   While you are bathing Mrs Stuart she becomes extremely upset and tearful. What would be your response?
7   One of the aims of care is to help Mrs Stuart to walk again. How might the nurse plan to do this?
8   Mr Stuart visits his wife frequently and on one visit asks how he may help with his wife's rehabilitation. What would be your response?

Two months later Mrs Stuart is ready to be discharged home. She is walking with the aid of a tripod. She still has a degree of paralysis in her right arm. Her speech is a little slurred but intelligible.

9 What preparations and arrangements must be made in order to:
   (a) prevent any problems from occurring at home?
   (b) continue her rehabilitation?

4.2   Answers

1

Present condition
- Assess the colour and respiratory rate. Is she able to maintain her own airway?
- Record the temperature, pulse and blood pressure. Is there any infection present? Is there any hypertension or bradycardia (indicating raised intercranial pressure)?
- Assess the level of consciousness.
- Ascertain the degree of paralysis and dysphagia.

Past history There is a need to elicit the health of Mrs Stuart before her admission so that it can be determined how much she has been incapacitated by her stroke. For example:
1 How mobile was she?
2 What was her mental state before admission?
3 Is she hard of hearing?
4 How good is her sight?

Social history Can Mr Stuart manage on his own? Are there any relatives who could help him?

Past medical history Is there any condition that may concern this admission (e.g. hypertension)? Is there any condition and/or medication that it is important to know about (e.g. diabetes, steroid treatment)?

---

2   Identify a means of communication, e.g. picture cards, a call bell in easy reach. Position her bed in easy view of the nurses' station.
3   - Incontinence
    - Dysphagia
    - Problems with vision
    - Difficulty in chewing

4

Incontinence is caused by a disturbance in some of the impulses from the bladder to the brain that control micturition. Altered levels of consciousness may also mean that if the impulse reaches the brain it may not be recognized.

Dysphagia due to paralysis of the cranial nerves involved in swallowing (the glossopharyngeal and accessory nerves) on the side opposite the cerebral incident.

Visual problems are caused by damage to the optic nerve. The medial fibres of each optic nerve from the retina cross over at the optic chiasma to terminate in the opposite side of the brain. Because of this partial crossing, the visual area of the left cerebral hemisphere receives impressions from the outer side of the retina of the left eye and from the inner side of the retina of the right eye. Thus, any cerebral damage may cause partial blindness in which the patient can only see one half of the normal field of vision (hemianopia).

Difficulty in chewing results from damage to the facial and glossopharyngeal nerves. Also, half of the tongue and the cheek muscles are paralysed. This also makes drinking difficult, so the patient may dribble saliva from the paralysed side of her mouth.

5 Explain to him that a disturbance in the blood flow to his wife's brain has damaged some nerve cells. She will need to be in hospital for close observation as the amount of recovery varies in each patient. She will remain in bed for the first 48 hours when it is most likely that a recurrence may occur. After this time it is more possible to determine her progress.

6 Ask why she is crying. Explain that you appreciate her frustrations. Endeavour to find out the problem with pictures, signs, writing paper and a pencil.

7 First, help her to regain her balance, sitting in bed, then sitting on the edge of the bed.
- Progress to standing. Use a full-length mirror to correct leaning.
- Ensure that she wears low-heeled shoes.
- Finally, teach her to walk with the use of a Zimmer frame at first, progressing to a stick.
- Remind her of her paralysed limb so that it does not drag or become damaged.

8 Be encouraging. Suggest he spends a day on the ward helping with his wife's care and observing the physio-therapist and speech therapist.

9 (a) **Prevention of problems**
- Arrange a home visit with the occupational therapist to ensure that she can manage stairs and use the bathroom.
- Arrange any alterations (stair rail, rails in bathroom, toilet) via the medical social worker.
- Ensure that Mr Stuart can help his wife. If not, Meals-on-Wheels or a district nurse may need to be organized.

(b) **Rehabilitation**

Organize community physiotherapy and speech therapy. If this is not possible arrange transport for visits to these departments, preferably on the same day.

4.3   Shirley Ascot—a baby with Down's syndrome

Shirley is 5 months old and has Down's syndrome. She is the first baby of Mr and Mrs Ascot, who are both in their mid-thirties.

1   What may have been Mr and Mrs Ascot's feelings and reactions when Shirley was born?
2   Identify the members of the District Handicapped Team and the role they may play in Shirley's care.
3   What other support is available in the community to help the family cope?

Mr and Mrs Ascot bring Shirley to clinic regularly and are keen to develop her potential to the full.

4   What should they be told about the rate at which Shirley is likely to develop?
5   How can they best stimulate Shirley to encourage her to learn?
6   What advice can they be given regarding Shirley's:
    (a)   skin care?
    (b)   feeding during infancy?
7   What care and advice will they require before and during a second pregnancy?
8   What alternative facilities are there to support and care for Shirley when she reaches adulthood, and what opportunities may they offer her?

4.3   Answers

1   • Shock and disbelief
    • Sense of grief and loss of a normal baby
    • Feelings of inadequacy
    • Uncertainty about the future
    • Anger and hostility
    • Embarrassment about Shirley's appearance
    • Feelings of protectiveness towards Shirley
    • Rejection of Shirley

Mr and Mrs Ascot may have any or all of these reactions. The feelings may come and go and may diminish in time.

2   The establishment of the District Handicapped Team was recommended in 1976 by the Court Report. Its role was to coordinate services for children with special needs.
    The core members of the team are:
    • paediatrician
    • clinical medical officer
    • social worker
    • representative from the community nursing services (child health)
    They may be supported by:
    • child psychiatrist
    • occupational therapist (who probably won't be involved in Shirley's care until she is older)
    • speech therapist (who will also give advice regarding feeding difficulties, e.g. excessive dribbling)
    • clinical psychologist (who is involved in assessing Shirley and in planning intervention to increase independence.)
    The above personnel will provide and coordinate services until the child has reached an agreed age, when they are transferred to the care of the Community Mental Handicap Team. The roles of these two teams may vary in different regions.

3   • The Health visitor and general practitioner
    • Family support units. These may include short-stay services and day care, and some may offer a crisis intervention service.
    • Toy libraries and playgroups
    • Attendance allowance when Shirley is 2 years old
    • Down's Children's Association
    • Mencap
    • Riding for the Disabled
    • Holidays for the Disabled

4   In general, both mental and motor development will be slower than normal, but Shirley will be capable of making steady progress.

Charts are available to show the average age at which children with Down's syndrome attain milestones, and Mr and Mrs Ascot should be given one of these. As an example, Shirley may not begin to walk until she is 19 months old; her speech development may lag behind considerably.

It is important to emphasize that Shirley is an individual and that the ages given on the charts are only average.

A general decrease in IQ score occurs as age advances and is an expected occurrence.

The degree of environmental stimulation will influence Shirley's rate of development.

5   • Shirley needs a secure and loving environment.
    • She will require more time to learn each new skill than a normal child.
    • As she tends to learn by mimicking people, this should be encouraged—repetition aids learning.
    • A natural liking for music and a sense of rhythm should be utilized to develop motor coordination.
    • The normal stimulation of holding, cuddling, etc., that normal babies require should be provided.
    • Shirley should be involved in everyday activities and opportunities taken up for stimulation.
    • Play and games should take place and should involve other members of the family.

6   (a) Shirley's skin will have a tendency to be less elastic than that of a normal child and may be quite dry and rough. This tendency will increase with age. The skin easily becomes chapped.

The areas of dry skin can be treated with creams, use of non-drying soaps, gentle cleansers, etc. The scalp may be dry and a gentle shampoo should be used.

(b) Shirley may be more likely to vomit than other children. This is usually due to slackness of the stomach muscles. As the muscles strengthen, so the vomiting decreases. She may become allergic to milk and may need changes to her diet.

Feeding difficulties are usually due to immaturity and weakness of the swallowing and sucking reflexes. This is usually overcome in a few days. If difficulties arise when weaning begins, Mrs Ascot could try pressing the spoon gently down on the tongue and gently pressing the chin up. This will then cause the tongue to move backwards.

Mrs Ascot may have to alter the size of the spoon or the texture of the food until Shirley finally develops the required coordination.

Overfeeding should be avoided as Shirley may have a predisposition to obesity.

7   Mr and Mrs Ascot will undergo genetic counselling. This will involve:

- an explanation of the risk factors involved in another child being affected. Depending on the type of chromosomal abnormality, the condition may or may not be inherited.
- Information about amniocentesis, which can be performed during pregnancy, and the choices should it prove to be positive.
- A chance for Mr and Mrs Ascot to ask questions and discuss their decision with a trained counsellor. Following discussion it will be up to Mr and Mrs Ascot to make an informed decision.

Once pregnant, Mrs Ascot should attend clinic regularly and remain as healthy as possible. Amniocentesis cannot be done until at least 14 weeks into pregnancy and is usually not done until 16 weeks. The risk of an amniocentesis should be explained. Mr and Mrs Ascot will require considerable support while waiting for the results.

8   The range of facilities available to provide care for Shirley once she reaches adulthood will vary from area to area. In some cases there may not be many facilities. Facilities for care include:

- The Pathway Scheme, where an officer may organize a place in open industry
- adult training centres/day care facilities
- the possibility of provision for further education
- the Disablement Resettlement Officer, who may help to choose suitable places for employment
- group homes for residential care, which are usually restricted due to lack of resources

5 Care of the Patient with Problems of Bones and Joints

5.1   Mr Smart—a man who is to undergo an amputation

Mr Charles Smart, aged 63 years, has been admitted to your ward with a gangrenous big toe on his right foot. Mr Smart has been a diabetic controlled with insulin for some years.

Six weeks ago Mr Smart dropped a hammer on his right big toe. At first the toe nail went black, but gradually the pain worsened and the whole toe became black. It has been decided to perform a below-knee amputation. Mr Smart lives in a semi-detached house with his wife.

1   What *specific* information will be required from Mr Smart on admission? Why will this information be useful?
2   What psychological preparation will Mr Smart need before surgery?
3   Describe Mr Smart's physical preparation for theatre.
4   Describe the management of Mr Smart's diabetes in the pre-operative and immediate post-operative period.
5   Describe the nursing measures that may be implemented to prevent contractures in Mr Smart's stump.
6   Explain the phenomenon of phantom pain.
7   What is the role of the physiotherapist in Mr Smart's rehabilitation?
8   Explain the preparation that will be required before Mr Smart's discharge home.
9   What advice should Mr Smart be given on discharge regarding:
(a) bandaging his stump?
(b) protection of his stump?
10   How may gangrene be prevented in diabetic patients?

5.1 Answers

1

Management of diabetes Check Mr Smart's dietary control, type of insulin used and dosages required. This is also an opportunity to assess his knowledge of his diabetes. Further education/stabilization can be given if necessary.

Home situation Assess the need for help on discharge and alterations/aids needed in the home. It is likely that Mr Smart will be in a wheelchair on discharge, awaiting artificial limb fitting. Can his bed be easily moved into a downstairs room? Is his wife well and able to help her husband?

Emotional state How do Mr and Mrs Smart feel about Mr Smart's forthcoming surgery?

Pain How much pain is Mr Smart experiencing? What does he find most helpful in relieving it? Is it affecting his daily activities? Does anything make it worse?

General condition Does Mr Smart seem at all breathless? How fit was he before gangrene affected his foot? Is he a heavy smoker?
   If his general condition is normally poor it may not be realistic to plan for an artificial limb. Any chronic chest or cardiac condition may be exacerbated by a general anaesthetic and/or heavy smoking.

---

2 Patients vary in their reaction to amputation according to their age and their intellectual, emotional and socio-economic status.

As well as feeling depressed, Mr Smart may feel angry that his diabetes has been the cause of losing his leg, especially if he has taken good care of his feet and diet.

The nurse should be available to let Mr Smart talk about his feelings. She should explain to him what he should expect following the operation. While it is important for her to be positive about Mr Smart's future, she should not be over-cheerful. Optimism may make Mr Smart think he should be brave and cheerful, and this may prevent him from revealing his true feelings. If it is possible, an amputee of similar age and lifestyle to Mr Smart who is managing successfully can visit.

3

Vital signs   A baseline should be recorded to compare with the post-operative condition.

Urinalysis   This should be performed to check renal function.

Diet   Ensure a high protein diet with at least 2 litres of fluid per day. This will ensure that the patient is in a good nutritional state to withstand the surgery and to help wound healing.

Exercise   The physiotherapist will teach Mr Smart exercises to strengthen his arm muscles. His three unaffected limbs can be put through the normal range of movements.
   A 'monkey-pole' can be attached to the bedhead to help with exercise. Deep breathing exercises can also be practised to avoid post-operative chest complications. If Mr Smart smokes, he will be advised to stop.

Nil-by-mouth   This should be the procedure 4–6 hours pre-operatively to avoid inhalation of vomit under anaesthesia.

Preparation for theatre   Mr Smart must be washed and dressed in a theatre gown and cap. Prostheses should be removed and any valuables put into safe keeping. He must be given a name band.

Pre-medication   This should be given 1 hour before theatre to dry up secretions and allay anxiety.

---

4   • **The pre-operative period** Mr Smart will be given a sliding scale of insulin during the pre-operative period as the infection of his foot will render his diabetes out of control.
   On the day of surgery he will be given his insulin as prescribed, but instead of breakfast, an infusion of dextrose/saline will be set up. At the time of his pre-medication, his blood sugar level will be measured to assess control.
   • **The post-operative period** The infusion will continue post-operatively until Mr Smart can eat and drink normally. Blood sugar levels will be measured every 3–4 hours and his insulin dose adjusted accordingly.

5   • The stump of the amputated limb must be kept in extension alignment with the body.
   • If possible, once the immediate post-operative period has passed, Mr Smart should be positioned prone for at least 1 hour daily.
   • The mattress must be firm to prevent a flexion contracture.

- Mr Smart should be encouraged to exercise the stump. He should practise flexing and extending his knee to prevent a flexion contraction of his right hip, and he should put the limb through the full range of movement while sitting on the edge of the bed.
- No pillows or sandbags should be placed around the stump as these could cause flexion contractures.

6   Phantom limb sensation is the sensation of experiencing the presence of the amputated limb. This is a normal, frequently occurring physiological response following amputation. Mr Smart should be warned of this feeling post-operatively and reassured that it is quite a normal experience.

Phantom limb pain is a more serious problem which may affect the patient's emotional acceptance of the amputation and his ability to use a prosthesis. Psychologists believe that this sensation of pain in a limb that has been amputated is an expression of the patient's grief or anxiety about the surgery, which he has not been able to express verbally. Thus it is important to give the patient an opportunity to reveal his feelings in the pre-operative period.

Phantom pain can be very disturbing for the patient, and adequate analgesia must be given. Reassurance that these pains and sensations will disappear eventually will also help the patient.

7   About 24 hours post-operatively the physiotherapist will visit the patient to initially help him regain his balance in the sitting position. The patient can be up for short periods in a wheelchair with a stump board under the knee. The physiotherapist can then begin to teach Mr Smart to transfer from the bed to the chair safely.

Mr Smart will not be allowed to put full weight on his stump until 6 weeks after surgery. (Deep tissues will take at least 6 weeks to form a firm scar.) Meanwhile, the physiotherapist can teach the patient to support himself on crutches or between parallel bars.

The physiotherapist will also ensure that Mr Smart maintains good muscle tone in his arms and remaining leg. Arm and shoulder exercises will be taught and Mr Smart will be encouraged to exercise his left leg by going through the full range of movements. Possible foot drop must be avoided by ankle exercises.

To maintain full range of movement in Mr Smart's right hip and knee and to build up strength in these muscles, passive exercises will be carried out initially. As soon as Mr Smart is able, he can perform active exercises. This will ensure that maximum ability is reached by the time his prosthesis can be fitted.

8
- Mrs Smart should be encouraged to visit during the day (if she is able) to see Mr Smart's care. She can then see the exercises he has been taught. She can also learn how to help him from the bed to the chair, and to the toilet and bath.
- The occupational therapist will visit Mr and Mrs Smart's home with the couple and the physiotherapist. They will assess the home for alteration(s) and/or aids needed. If necessary, rails will be fitted and the bedroom moved downstairs.
- The nurse should check that Mr Smart's diabetes is re-stabilized and that he and his wife have a good understanding of this condition.

9
(a) **Bandaging** Mr and Mrs Smart should both be shown how to apply Mr Smart's stump bandage. The stump is usually bandaged with an over-and-under method initially and then with spiral turns. All parts of the bandaged limb should be equally compressed to help the stump shrink and to shape it for wearing a prosthesis.

The bandage should be changed at least twice a day. If Mr Smart perspires a lot, the stump should be washed and dried before applying the new bandage.

He should be advised to wash the bandages between wearings, rinsing them well. To maintain their elasticity they should be dried flat, and when dry, rolled without stretching them.

(b) **Protection of the stump** Mr Smart must be aware that to knock his stump or to injure it in any way may cause a breakdown of the wound.

He should observe the stump for irritation or redness caused by incorrect bandaging. He should allow the stump to return to normal before reapplying the bandage.

He should be particularly careful when moving from the chair to the bed not to knock his stump.

Torn or stretched stump socks must be thrown away—a darn or crease could cause ulceration of his stump.

10
- The feet should be bathed and dried well every day.
- Toe-nails should be trimmed straight across. Any other foot care should be performed by a chiropodist.
- The feet should be inspected daily for soreness, infection or calluses. Any abnormality should be reported.
- Shoes and socks should be well fitting.
- Socks should not be rough or darned.

- Diet and insulin dose should be balanced.
- If the patient suffers pins and needles in his feet, he should inform his doctor.

5.2   Mrs Kelly—an elderly lady with a fractured femur

Mrs Elizabeth Kelly, aged 72 years, slipped on some wet leaves while on her way to the local shops and broke her leg. An ambulance was called and she was brought to the accident and emergency department.

Mrs Kelly lives with her unmarried daughter and is an active member of the community. She is secretary of the Women's Institute and does voluntary work at the local hospital.

1   State the aims of first aid treatment and describe how you would achieve these aims as the person finding Mrs Kelly.

A fractured neck of femur is diagnosed and Mrs Kelly is transferred to the orthopaedic ward. She is pale, cold and clammy, and trembling. Her pulse is fast and thready and her blood pressure is low.

2   Explain the reasons for Mrs Kelly's physical condition.
3   Describe the nursing care that may be implemented to relieve these symptoms.

Mrs Kelly has her fractured leg put into skin traction until she is fit for surgery. The insertion of a Smith-Petersen nail is planned for 2 days time.

4   Mrs Kelly's daughter asks you why her mother needs an operation. A young colleague of hers was treated only with traction when he broke his hip in a motor-bike accident. What will you reply?
5   Explain the purpose and principles of skin traction.
6   What care will Mrs Kelly require in relation to her skin traction?
7   Outline the *specific* nursing care Mrs Kelly will need in preparation for theatre.

Mrs Kelly returns from theatre following an internal fixation. She has an intravenous infusion in progress and one suction drain in an anterior wound.

8 Explain to a junior colleague the care of Mrs Kelly's drain.
9 Describe Mrs Kelly's remobilization.

5.2 Answers

1 The aims of first aid are:
   • to sustain life
   • to prevent the patient's condition becoming worse
   • to promote recovery
   These can be achieved in Mrs Kelly's case in the following ways:

To sustain life
• Ensure that Mrs Kelly is in no danger from further injury due to traffic.
• Treat any asphyxia, haemorrhage or severe wound.

To prevent the condition worsening
• Do not move unless necessary.
• Steady and support the injured part.
• Reassure Mrs Kelly that you are a nurse and that help is on the way.
• Keep Mrs Kelly as comfortable as possible.
• Monitor her pulse, colour, respirations and level of consciousness.

To promote recovery
• Call an ambulance (or ask a passer-by to do so)

---

2 There may be considerable blood loss from a fractured femur into the surrounding tissues. Loss of blood from the circulation causes the heart to beat faster to compensate for the loss. The pulse will therefore be fast. It is thready because less blood is being pumped around the body. This reduced cardiac output causes a fall in the systolic blood pressure.

The body also compensates for blood loss by vasoconstriction in the peripheral blood vessels to direct blood to more vital organs. Ischaemia causes the skin to become pale and cold.

These features of hypovolaemic shock may be exacerbated by pain and anxiety. Such emotions interfere with normal control of the blood vessels by the autonomic nervous system. Stimulation of the sympathetic nervous system further constricts peripheral blood vessels and increases activity of the sweat glands, resulting in a clammy feel to the skin. Sympathetic stimulation also dilates major vessels to alter the pulse and blood pressure as described above.

3   The nurse should be sure to relieve Mrs Kelly's pain and fear to avoid exacerbating her hypovolaemic shock.

Analgesia (e.g. dihydrocodeine 30–60 mg 4–6 hourly) must be given as required. Mrs Kelly should be handled gently and as little as possible to avoid causing her further pain.

A competent and reassuring manner will help to allay Mrs Kelly's anxiety. She should be given explanations of what is happening to her. The presence of her daughter may also help to reassure her.

A blood transfusion will be prescribed to replace blood loss. Nursing care will involve ensuring that the transfusion runs at the rate prescribed. Observation of her pulse and blood pressure will be taken $\frac{1}{2}$–1 hourly to monitor her condition. Any further reduction in blood pressure or increase in pulse must be reported.

4   Explain to Mrs Kelly's daughter that the treatment of broken limbs varies according to the site of the injury and the age of the patient.

Explain that treatment by traction can take about 12 weeks until the bone has healed. Although her mother is fairly fit and healthy, that amount of time confined to bed at her age is not advisable as so many complications can occur (e.g. bed sores, chest infection or clotting of the blood in the affected leg).

Surgery, on the other hand, means that Mrs Kelly can start to get out of bed the day afterwards.

Also, Mrs Kelly's injury is at the neck of the femur which is a difficult site to realign by traction. In younger adults, whose bones are harder, the break is usually in the shaft of the bone. [Diagrams may help to illustrate this (Fig. 5)].

Also, a break at this point in the femur, unless repaired early, can interfere with the blood supply to the head of the femur leading to the death of the bone.

5   Traction is a steady pull on a part of the body and is used to reduce and immobilize fractures to overcome muscle spasm, to stretch adhesions, and to correct deformity.

Skin traction is achieved in elderly patients by applying wide bands of latex foam rubber with a strong cloth back (zentfoam) to avoid damaging fragile skin. Weights are applied to these bands so that the pull of the weights is transmitted directly to the involved bone. The foot of Mrs Kelly's bed will be elevated so that her body will provide countertraction and will keep her leg in alignment without shortening the limb.

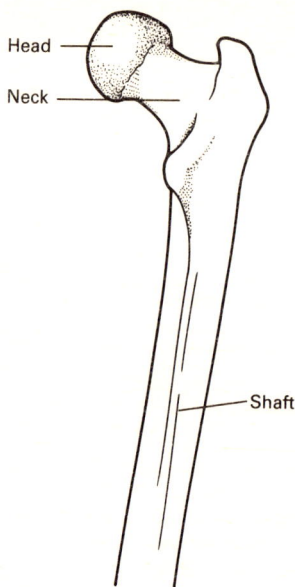

Fig. 5   The femur

6   • Examine Mrs Kelly's skin for evidence of pressure or
       friction on the knees or ankles due directly to the traction.
     • Check also her buttocks and elbows for signs of soreness.
     • Observe for features of deep vein thrombosis (swelling,
       redness, cramp-like pain in the calves) due to inactivity
       or pressure on the popliteal vessels.
     • Check the traction apparatus to ensure that the weights
       are hanging freely above the floor and that the ropes are
       running freely through the pulleys.
     • Check the position of Mrs Kelly's leg. The traction should
       correct the external rotation caused by the fracture.
     • Explain to Mrs Kelly the purpose of the equipment and
       that she can still move herself in the bed to change her
       position. She will not be able to sit upright or lie com-
       pletely on one side as this will prevent the traction from
       being effective.

7

Assessment of her general condition Does she appear 'chesty'? Is her skin intact and healthy? Is she pyrexial? (Any abnormalities should be treated before surgery.)

Urinalysis It is particularly important before this type of surgery to ensure that Mrs Kelly does not have a urinary tract infection. Because of the wound site, a urine infection can contaminate the operated area.

Leg exercises Mrs Kelly should be encouraged to exercise her good leg to enable her to mobilize as soon as possible post-operatively. Stretching exercises will help to prevent a post-operative chest infection. This is a specific problem due to Mrs Kelly's age and the fact that she cannot sit upright due to the traction.

---

8   Initially, the junior nurse's knowledge about suction drains should be checked. She will need to appreciate that these drains reach deeply into the wound, sucking out drainage to prevent a haematoma.

It is important to check the drain to ensure that a vacuum is present in the bottle, or the apparatus will not function. (The method of checking will vary according to the type of suction drain used—you should know the type used in your hospital.)

Drainage should be observed $\frac{1}{2}$-hourly immediately after surgery, and any excess bleeding must be reported. The amount of drainage should be measured at least daily when the drain is changed. The amount and characteristic of the drainage should be recorded on the fluid chart.

The drain is removed, using an aseptic technique, when drainage has ceased or is minimal (usually 48 hours after surgery).

While the drain is in situ the tubing should not be kinked. Mrs Kelly should be reminded about the drain, especially when up in the chair, so that she does not pull upon the tubing.

9   If her condition is otherwise satisfactory, Mrs Kelly can get up in the chair the day after surgery. She should put her weight on her good leg at this stage. Non-weight-bearing leg exercises can be encouraged at this stage to prevent muscle wastage and stiffness.

As the wound is over a large weight-bearing joint, the sutures will not be removed for 10–14 days. Once they have been removed, weight-bearing with a walking aid can commence.

5.3 Mr Barber—a young man with fractures of the tibia and fibula

Peter Barber, aged 24 years, is a single West Indian man who works as a dispatch rider with a courier service in the centre of London. He has been admitted to the accident and emergency department after a road traffic accident. His motor-bike went out of control on a patch of grease when going round a right-hand bend. He has sustained a compound fracture of his right tibia and fibula.

1 Describe, giving reasons, Peter's care and treatment in the accident and emergency department.
2 During his stay in the department, Peter is given an injection of tetanus toxoid. Explain:
   (a) why this is necessary
   (b) the action of tetanus toxoid
3 Explain to a junior colleague the reason for Peter's features on admission.

Peter is transferred from the accident and emergency department to theatre for an open reduction of his fracture. He returns to the orthopaedic ward with a full-length plaster of Paris cast on his right leg. A window has been cut in the plaster over his leg wound.

4 Explain how the nurse will observe for post-operative respiratory problems in patients of Peter's colour.
5 Describe the initial care of Peter's leg while it is in plaster.
6 Describe the care and management of Peter's wound.
7 Explain how the knowledge of the healing of fractures can be used to plan Peter's care.
8 What actions and exercises will Peter be encouraged to practise while his leg is immobilized?
9 Before discharge, Peter asks about the removal of his plaster. What advice can he be given?

5.3   Answers

1   • **Care of shock** Peter should be given analgesia as soon as possible once a head injury has been discounted. (Your answer should include an example, e.g. intramuscular papaveretum 15–20 mg.) He should be reassured by explaining what will happen to him.

He should only be moved if absolutely necessary and his leg should be kept immobilized (either by use of the ambulanceman's inflatable splint or sandbags) to minimize pain and shock.

If blood loss has been a problem, intravenous fluids must be given, to be followed by a blood transfusion after the blood has been taken for grouping and cross-matching. The infusion must be regulated as prescribed. A fluid chart should be kept, particularly noting urine output, as prolonged hypotension may cause acute renal failure.

Shock should be monitored by half-hourly observation of the pulse and blood pressure. Any further tachycardia or hypotension must be reported.

   • **Treatment** Baseline observations of temperature, pulse, respirations and blood pressure will be taken when Peter is first admitted.

He will be observed for any injuries other than the compound fracture. Information gathered from the ambulancemen may reveal the likelihood of a head injury, or they may have noted other injuries in their initial examination.

A sedative will not be necessary if analgesia has been administered within the last 4 hours.

2   (a) Peter has a compound fracture which means that he has an open wound. As his wound was sustained in dirty conditions—a road surface which has been contaminated by all sorts of vehicles—he is at risk of developing tetanus. *Clostridium tetani*, the causative organism, is an anaerobic bacillus found especially in manured soils. Unless Peter has had a course of tetanus toxoid within the last 2 years it is preferable to increase his immunity at this time of increased risk.

(b) Active immunity to disease by immunization takes some months to establish. Peter is provided with tetanus toxoid either as an initial immunizing dose or as a booster for previous immunization.

Tetanus toxoid consists of a modified toxin to stimulate the production of antibodies against *Clostridium tetani*.

3 Ask the junior nurse what features can be demonstrated by a patient with a fracture. She should be able to list pain, loss of function, deformity, swelling and shortening. You can then explain these features as follows:

Deformity and shortening	For 10–40 minutes after a fracture the muscles surrounding the bone are flaccid. Then they go into spasm, causing deformity and shortening.
Swelling	When the bone breaks, the local periosteum and surrounding blood vessels are torn. The tissue surrounding the fracture swells due to internal bleeding and inflammatory exudate.
Loss of function	Instability of the broken bone and pain lead to inability to use the limb.
Pain	Broken bone causes severe pain. As explained above it is not only the bone that is injured.

4 A certain amount of pallor can be detected in the face of a coloured person, but an additional check should be made for pallor of the fingernails and the mucous membrane linings of the lips, mouth and inner sides of the lower eyelids. These should be a pink colour in a healthy person, regardless of race.

5 On return from theatre Peter's leg should be elevated on pillows for the next 24 hours to prevent swelling of the traumatized limb, which may cause the plaster to become too tight. His leg should be exposed to the atmosphere to aid drying of the plaster. This can be achieved by the use of a cradle.

During the first 48 hours after the application of the plaster, Peter's leg must be observed, initially every half-hour, for any signs that the plaster is too tight. Warning signs are:
- pain
- paraesthesia
- pallor of toes
- foot in plaster colder than other foot

- pulse reduced or absent in the foot
- power loss
- swelling of toes

Any of these should be reported immediately as the plaster may have to be split or removed.

Until Peter has become accustomed to the weight of the plaster, the nurse should lift his leg for him. Until the plaster is completely dry it must be held in the palm of the hand to avoid indentations.

It is also important to observe for any indications of a plaster sore developing. Any complaints of itching, tingling, burning or severe pain under the plaster should be investigated. Undue heat may be felt under the plaster by the patient and on the outside of the cast by the nurse. Any unexplained pyrexia could also be caused by the presence of a plaster sore.

6 Compound fractures, especially when sustained in dirty environments, always carry the risk of osteomyelitis. For this reason the wound and surrounding skin are washed with a mild antiseptic in theatre. To loosen and remove earth, dirt or blood, dilute hydrogen peroxide is used with a scrubbing brush. The surgeon will then put on a fresh gown and glove to further clean the operative area.

The wound is left open to drain and a window left in the plaster to allow easy access.

The wound is dressed as necessary using an aseptic technique. It should be observed for healing by contracture and granulation. Any tissue necrosis should be carefully removed.

A diagram is kept on the care plan to illustrate the stage of progress of the wound.

The wound is also observed for infection. Any inflammation, discharge or complaints from Peter of heat or pain in the wound should be reported.

If the wound is draining, care should be taken to ensure that the dressing is changed as often as necessary to keep it dry.

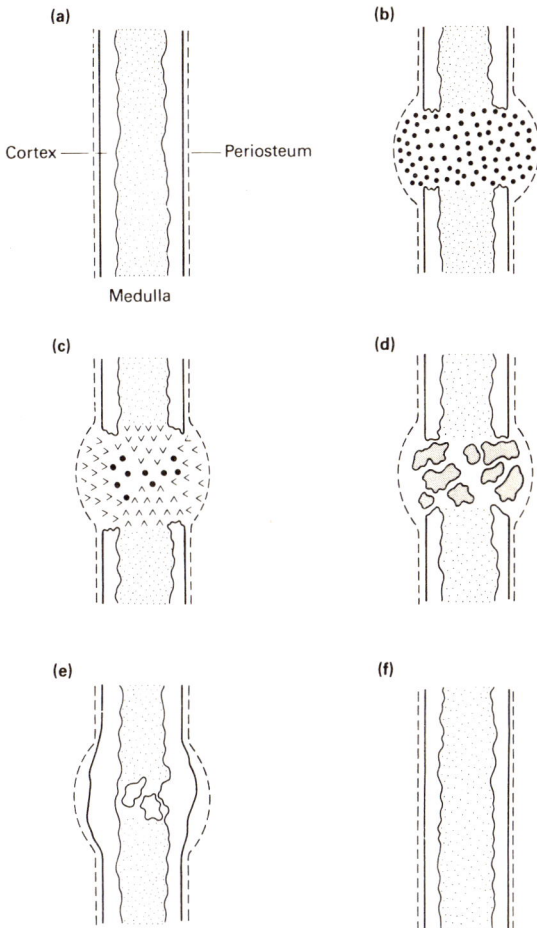

Fig. 6 Stages in the healing of fractures in long bones. (a) Anatomy of long bone. (b) Fracture leads to bleeding from severed vessels. Blood clot accumulates in the gap and elevation of the periosteum occurs. This is followed by a brisk inflammatory reaction. (c) Granulation tissue is formed. (d) Osteoid and cartilage appear. This is known as the 'provisional callus'. (e) The callus is replaced by new lamellar bone. The ends are now firmly united. (f) The new lamellar bone is remodelled.

7   See Fig. 6.

Summary of fracture healing	Patient need	Related care
Clot formation	Keep limb immobilized	Maintain immobilization of limb in correct alignment
Formation of blood supply	Good blood supply to affected part	Ensure that the circulation is not impaired after reduction of the fracture. Observe the affected limb for bleeding or infection.
Osteoid tissue	Healing of bone	Provide high calcium, vitamin D and protein diet.
Osteocyte activity	Alignment of healed limb	Ensure that the limb is maintained in correct alignment.
Union of fracture	Prevention of refracture or dislocation when cast is removed	Help the patient during his first use of the limb after removal of the plaster. Provide support for joints immobilized by the cast.

8   Peter should be allowed to sit out of bed as soon as possible, with the affected limb elevated on a stool at all times.

When his wound has healed, providing the fracture is stable, he can commence walking with crutches with the physiotherapist. Until this point he will be encouraged to exercise his unaffected limb and arms to strengthen these muscles as, at first, he will be either partially or non-weight-bearing with crutches.

The physiotherapist will show him how to strengthen his arm muscles by using a chest expander and by lifting himself up with the use of a monkey-pole. The left leg can be strengthened by straight leg exercises as well as by putting the leg through a full range of movements.

He should also move the toes of his affected leg.

9   Ask him exactly what he wishes to know. He will need to know that he will have to retain his plaster for about 16 weeks.

It will be removed with an electric saw but Peter should be reassured that it is a vibrating instrument, not a cutting one. If plaster shears are also used, these have a flat under-surface to the cutting edge to protect the limb.

Because his leg will have been immobilized for so long, it will be stiff and will need to be gradually strengthened by exercises which the physiotherapist will show him. Sudden or strenuous movements must be avoided when the plaster is first removed as these could be very painful.

Peter may find that his leg is very dry after months in plaster. Baby oil or arachis oil will soon help tc moisten the skin. His leg will also look very thin due to muscle wasting. This will soon be remedied by exercise.

5.4   Miss James—a woman undergoing a laminectomy

Miss Penny James, aged 38 years, is a community nurse. Six months ago she felt a sudden pain in her lower back while lifting an elderly, obese patient. Her general practitioner diagnosed a prolapsed intervertebral disc and prescribed conservative treatment.

Six months later her condition has not improved and she has been admitted for a myelogram and surgery.

1   With reference to anatomy and physiology explain Miss James' condition to a junior nurse.
2   What specific information will you need during Miss James' assessment in order to plan her care?
3   Bearing in mind that Miss James has been out of general nursing for 14 years, how will you explain the myelogram to her?

After the myelogram the surgeons decide to perform a laminectomy.

4   Describe, giving reasons, the post-operative observations you will carry out on Miss James on her return from theatre.
5   Explain how the nurse can keep Miss James' spine in alignment post-operatively.
6   Describe how Miss James can be best helped to eat and drink before she can get out of bed.
7   What advice will be given to Miss James before her discharge?
8   Discuss the prevention of back injury for nurses.

5.4   Answers

1   Ask the junior nurse about her present knowledge of prolapsed discs. Ask her what she thinks will happen if an
intervertebral disc slips out of position.

Having discussed this show her a diagram, as below, to
illustrate your explanation.

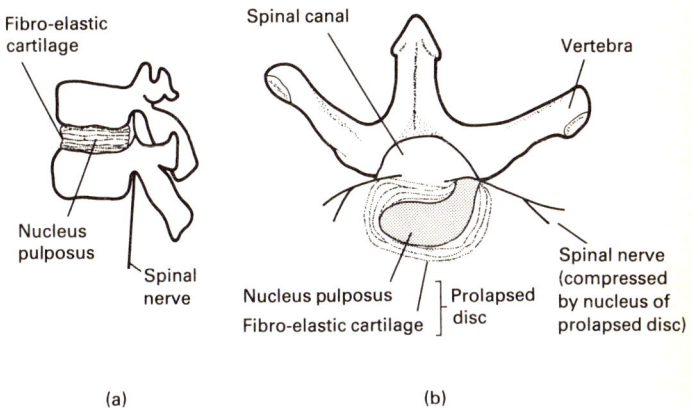

Fig. 7   (a) Normal disc (lateral view). (b) Prolapsed disc (anterior view).

Each intervertebral disc is made up of an outer ring of
fibrocartilage and an inner mass of elastic, soft tissue,
nucleus pulposus. The discs are situated between the bodies
of adjacent vertebrae where they act as 'shock absorbers'.

Prolapse of an intervertebral disc is usually the result of
injury or prolonged strain. The nucleus pulposus ruptures
out of the surrounding fibrocartilage. If the prolapse is large
it may herniate into the spinal cord and compress one of
the spinal nerves, causing pain and sometimes impairment
of the sensory and motor function of that part.

2

Mobility
How much has Miss James' mobility been affected by her injury?
What activity or position eases or aggravates her pain?

Elimination
Has Miss James' bowel and bladder function been affected by her
prolapsed disc?

Sleeping
Does pain interfere with Miss James' sleep?
What does she usually do to get back to sleep?

Understanding
How much does Miss James know about the condition and her proposed treatment? (You should not presume that because she is a nurse, she will not need reassurance or explanations.)

3 Ask Miss James what she knows about a myelogram so that you can build on her present knowledge and correct any misconceptions

She will need to know that a myelogram consists of injecting a radiopaque substance into the spinal canal. Any abnormalities of the spinal canal such as a prolapsed intervertebral disc which herniates into the canal can then be demonstrated by X-ray films.

She will not need any special preparation for this investigation other than wearing a theatre gown for easy access to her spine. In the X-ray department she will be required to lie on her side with her knees drawn up to her chest and her head drawn down to her knees. She will be asked to remain as still as possible during the procedure as movement may cause injury. A local anaesthetic will be injected into the lumbar region to prevent pain when the spinal needle is inserted. Once the dye has been injected through the spinal needle, the X-ray table may be tilted to enable the dye to flow up and down the spinal canal, and X-rays are taken. When sufficient films have been taken the dye is removed by movement of the spinal needle, which may cause some slight discomfort. However, a nurse will remain with Miss James to help her maintain this position and to reassure her.

After the procedure she will return to the ward where she will be asked to lie flat in bed for 12–24 hours to minimize the likelihood of headache. She should not be afraid to call for a nurse should she require anything or if she should develop any pain.

4

Potential problem	Observations
Potential asphyxia due to inhalation of vomit or secretions	Observe Miss James' colour and respirations. Report any dyspnoea, pallor and cyanosis, which may indicate an obstructed airway.

Potential cord compression due to oedema or haemorrhage	Take half-hourly measurements of pulse and blood pressure. Report any tachycardia or hypotension. Observe the wound site for any swelling or leakage of cerebro-spinal fluid or blood. Assess Miss James' sensory and motor function by: • asking her to move her legs • checking her ability to feel sensation along her legs. Report any impairment. Check when Miss James first passes urine (urine retention may be due to cord compression)

5   As Miss James has a spinal wound it is important to keep her spine in alignment in order to promote healing.

Immediately after surgery she should be positioned supine with her head to one side for 4–6 hours. After this time she can be turned 'log fashion'. To do this the patient should put her arms straight by her side and make herself as stiff as a log. Then the nurse can roll her over in this position.

Miss James should not lift her hips to sit on the bedpan. A slipper bedpan should be used, onto which she can roll. Pillows can then be placed under her back to support her.

Miss James' locker and belongings should be left within easy reach so that she does not have to stretch to get anything she needs.

6   Eating and drinking will be difficult for Miss James while she is confined to bed and lying flat.

Easily digestible foods should be advised to avoid indigestion. Small meals will also be better tolerated in this position.

Her food will have to be cut up for her and she may need help in feeding herself. Flexi-straws will facilitate drinking in this awkward position.

Diet should consist of roughage such as bran added to cereals, fresh fruit and vegetables to overcome the problem of constipation which is likely to occur during a period of comparative immobility. A daily fluid intake of 2–3 litres should be encouraged to also help prevent constipation.

7 Miss James should avoid wearing high-heeled shoes which throw the body's centre of gravity out of alignment and cause back strain. She should instead wear shoes with only a moderately-sized heel which give her feet good support.

Slippers should not be worn for long periods of time as they do not provide adequate support.

Miss James should be aware of her posture when sitting and standing. She should always sit upright, preferably in an upright chair rather than an easy chair.

Exercise should be encouraged to strengthen the back muscles and maintain a good posture. Swimming is a useful exercise for strengthening muscles.

The following reminders should be given about the principles of lifting:

- Bend the knees, not the back.
- Do not perform any heavy lifting (i.e. no more than a full kettle for the next 6 weeks).
- Lift objects close to the body.

Miss James should remain off work for at least 12 weeks when her condition will be reassessed.

8 Back injury amongst nurses is common—59% of nurses have suffered back pain, 70% of these cases being due to lifting [Lloyd, F. G. & Breen, A. C. (1979) *A Study of Back Pain in Nurses*. Presented to the Society for Back Pain Research, London].

All nurses should be shown correct posture and exercises to strengthen their back muscles. They should be taught how to lift in their introductory course and should not be allowed to lift patients until they have been taught to do so properly.

They should be taught the principles of lifting as follows:

- to bend at the knees rather than at the waist
- to lift close to the body
- to use mechanical lifting aids whenever possible

They should be taught never to lift patients on their own and to use as many nurses as necessary. One nurse should take charge and plan and coordinate the lift.

However, such guides are difficult to follow in certain instances. A nurse may be left alone during meal breaks on night-duty, with no-one to help her to lift. Community nurses are often alone and working with low beds and cramped situations. In some hospitals hoists are not available on every ward.

Recent research [Rogers, S. (January, 1985) *Nursing Times*, **81** (3)] has shown that although nurses are taught lifting in their introductory course they do not have enough time to practise these skills. This paper also reveals that what is taught is not practised on the ward, which seems to indicate that more time should be allocated to teaching lifting, both in the introductory course and at regular intervals during basic and post-basic training.

5.5 Alan Harris—a young adult undergoing a meniscectomy

Alan Harris, aged 21 years, a shop assistant, has been admitted to the ward for a meniscectomy. He was first seen in the accident and emergency department last week following an injury to his right knee during a football match. On this occasion he was unable to walk and his right knee was swollen and painful. His knee was locked and he could not extend his leg. A diagnosis of torn meniscus was made. This admission was arranged so that surgery could correct the injury and prevent permanent disability.

On admission Alan seems very confident and talkative. He is, however, concerned about his future with regard to sport.

1 List the information Alan will require on admission and before surgery.
2 How would you explain Alan's condition to a junior colleague?
3 Describe Alan's specific pre-operative care.
4 What are the responsibilities of the nurse taking Alan to theatre?

Alan returns from theatre following removal of his right medial meniscus. The cruciate ligaments and joint surfaces were checked but found to be normal. His leg is immobilized.

5 Give the three ways in which Alan's leg may be immobilized post-operatively.
6 Haemoarthrosis and synovial effusion are specific potential problems of this type of surgery. Explain these complications and plan the care needed to reduce their incidence.
7 The quadriceps muscle wastes rapidly when not functioning. How can Alan be helped to regain his muscle tone post-operatively?
8 What advice should Alan be given on discharge?
9 Discuss the specific points to consider when caring for a young adult such as Alan.

5.5 Answers

1 • The date of surgery
   • His pre-operative preparation (see ans. **3**)
   • The ward lay-out and routine
   • Recognition of the staff and how to ring/call for help
   • The arrangements for visitors
   • What the surgery entails and the likely post-operative condition
   • An outline of post-operative remobilization—immobilization for 24 hours—standing with crutches—exercises as shown by the physiotherapist
   • Discharge after 1–7 days (according to the individual surgeon/hospital)
   • Advice regarding his job (off for 3–4 weeks)
   • Advice regarding sport (football should be possible again provided that Alan is conscientious with his exercises post-operatively)

2 A twisting movement of the knee while the knee is flexed and the foot is flat on the ground can cause a torn meniscus. It is a common injury in football and skiing, where such movement is common.

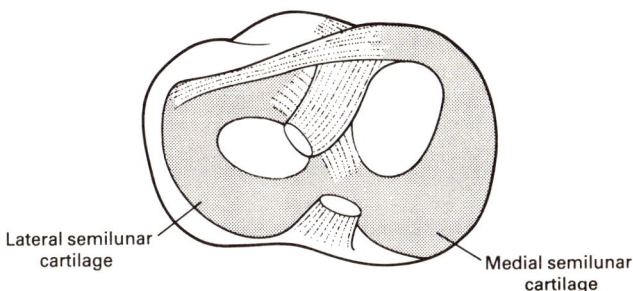

Fig. 8 Superior surface of the tibia.

Lateral semilunar cartilage

Medial semilunar cartilage

The menisci are two semilunar cartilage pads attached to the top of the tibia. They act as shock absorbers.

A torn meniscus may cause pain, swelling and tenderness in the joint. The patient may complain of clicking or snapping sensations during activity. If the torn meniscus becomes displaced the knee may become 'locked' as the cartilage becomes jammed between the femur and the tibia.

3 **Physiotherapy** Alan must be taught breathing exercises to

prevent chest infection and deep vein thrombosis. The use of a tourniquet during surgery together with immobilization of the limb post-operatively make clotting episodes a particular complication.

Alan can also be told about the importance of learning quadriceps drill (see ans. 7) and practising it after surgery. He can also be shown how to use crutches.

- **Skin preparation** is of particular importance in orthopaedic surgery to prevent infection leading to osteomyelitis.

The affected leg will be shaved from the pubic area to the ankle. A full bath or shower is taken and the skin on the affected leg is then painted with povidone-iodine 2% (or some other example) from the surgery site outwards.

4
- To ensure that the pre-operative checklist has been completed (i.e. that notes and X-rays are available, the consent form is signed, pre-medication has been given and recorded, urinalysis and vital signs have been recorded, an identiband is present, and the prosthesis is removed)
- To check the patient's name and hospital number with the porter to ensure that the right patient has been collected
- To help the patient onto the trolley if necessary and to ensure that modesty is maintained.
- To provide emotional support and to explain the journey to theatre if it is lengthy (the patient is lying flat and cannot see around him)
- To stay with the patient in the anaesthetic room and to provide reassurance to promote relaxation; to explain any frightening events or remarks overheard from theatre staff
- To check the patient's name and hospital number with the anaesthetist to ensure that the correct patient has been received; to emphasize any allergies or concerns of the patient (e.g. inhaling gas)

5   Following meniscectomy the affected limb is immobilized to prevent swelling. It may be immobilized by:
- **Compression dressings**—firm crêpe bandage and wool *or* a Robert-Jones pressure bandage
- **Cylinder plaster of Paris**—a cast which does not extend over the ankle and foot and which is straight
- **Knee immobilizer**—a posterior splint of metal or plaster of Paris to augment a crêpe bandage. This holds the leg in extension and is more comfortable than a cylinder cast.

6

Problem	Aim	Care
Haemoarthrosis (Bleeding into the joint from large vessels)	Early detection	Observe for features—swelling, pain, malaise, loss of sensation. If such features occur the bandage or cast should be cut longitudinally and a fresh bandage applied with less tension.
Synovial effusion (fluid in the synovial space due to an inflammatory reaction following trauma of surgery)	Reduction of swelling	Elevate and support the leg. Observe for local discomfort and difficulty with exercising.

7 **Quadriceps drill**
As soon as Alan has regained consciousness he should be encouraged to carry out the following quadriceps exercises for 5 minutes every hour when awake:
- Tighten the quadriceps muscle by pulling the kneecap into the thigh or by pressing the back of the knee into the mattress.
- Move the toes.
- Perform straight leg raising. Initially this can be done by the nurse. The hand is placed under the patient's heel and the leg is raised to 60–90° hip flexion. The patient can then lower the leg himself. As the patient becomes more able he can do this independently and practise holding his leg in the air before lowering it.

8 Alan must expect 6–8 weeks of rehabilitation before regaining normal function.

He should continue with his exercises and attend knee classes and physiotherapy as an outpatient.

Mobilization of his leg can commence on the third/fourth day post-operatively when knee flexion exercises can begin.

He should attend the orthopaedic clinic in 2 weeks time for the removal of sutures and reassessment.

He may return to work in 3/4 weeks but should not kneel

for long periods initially. Some numbness is to be expected at first, but this does not mean that feeling has gone for good. (*Note* There may be variations in this part of the question. Hospitals vary and discharge can occur at any time from 48 hours to 10 days post-operatively.)

9

Anxiety The young adult is often keen to appear unconcerned and knowledgeable when he is actually quite worried. Alan's talkativeness on admission could be a feature of this. The nurse should be able to recognize hidden stress and provide appropriate support.

Flexibility Ward routine should not be rigid. Patients such as Alan are relatively healthy. They probably need less sleep than older and more ill patients. They probably also prefer to be allowed to sleep rather than to be woken early for a cup of tea.

Young adults find rigid rules irritating and may find ways of expressing rebelliousness, disturbing others in the ward. The nurse must rationalize rules and also give the young adult patient involvement in planning his own care so he does not feel that his independence has been completely lost.

Pain The young adult male may think that it is not manly to express pain. The nurse should be alert for non-verbal signals of pain and should suggest rather than offer, pain relief.

Activity Young, comparatively healthy adults have a lot of energy. They should be given the opportunity to channel this energy into physiotherapy. Ideally, they should be encouraged to be up and about during the day.

Their environment should provide interests of this age group, such as radio/cassette recorders, cards, snooker, etc.

Peer support is important as a young adult and it may be useful to situate such patients together in a group.

Nursing staff Young nurses of a similar age group to the young adult patient may find that they identify with the patient. The nurse may then find it difficult to maintain a professional relationship, which may cause difficulties when carrying out nursing care.

The older nurse may transfer some of his/her conflicts with his/her own adolescent children and may tend to become authoritarian. This may in turn cause rebellion in the young adult patient.

5.6   Mrs Edmunds—a woman with rheumatoid arthritis

Mrs Betty Edmunds, a 38-year-old housewife, has been admitted to your ward in an acute phase of rheumatoid arthritis. On admission she looks thin and tired. Her fingers are obviously swollen and deformed. Her temperature is 39°C.

It has been decided to rest Mrs Edmunds while she is in the acute phase of her illness. She has been prescribed indomethacin 50 mg three times a day, dihydrocodeine 30–60 mg 4–6 hourly as required, and ferrous sulphate 200 mg twice daily.

Mrs Edmunds lives in a three-bedroomed house with her husband, a long-distance lorry driver, and her two sons, aged 9 and 12 years.

1   What specific information will be required from Mrs Edmunds on admission in order to plan her care?
2   Describe the nursing actions that would enable Mrs Edmunds to rest.
3   Explain the differences between osteoarthritis and rheumatoid arthritis to a junior colleague.
4   Mr Edmunds asks you if the fact that their house is very cold and draughty has made his wife ill. What should you say?
5   Describe the nursing measures that can be taken to prevent the potential problem of limb deformity while Mrs Edmunds is confined to bed.
6   State the possible side-effects of Mrs Edmunds' drug therapy. How may their incidence be minimized?
7   When Mrs Edmunds' acute phase has subsided she will need help to regain muscle tone and joint mobility. Describe how this should be done.
8   What help and advice can be given to Mrs Edmunds and her family when she is ready for discharge?

5.6   Answers

1 • **Understanding** Assess Mrs Edmunds' understanding of her illness. Will education need to be part of your care?
   • **Emotional factors** Arthritis causes pain, deformity and reduced mobility. This can make the patient very anxious and depressed. Anxiety will increase muscle spasm and pain. Endeavour to discover how Mrs Edmunds feels about her condition.
   • **Pain** Ask Mrs Edmunds about the presence of pain and stiffness and the circumstances under which these are aggravated and relieved.
   • **Mobility** Discover the exact level of Mrs Edmunds' mobility and recent changes in this degree of movement.
   • **Family circumstances** Who is looking after the children if Mr Edmunds is away from home? If Mrs Edmunds is anxious about this, it may delay her recovery.
   • **Home life** Does Mrs Edmunds have any particular problems at home, either with dressing, bathing or with aspects of housework? These problems can then be tackled as soon as Mrs Edmunds is able to mobilize. Aids can be ordered immediately.
   • **Eating and drinking** Has Mrs Edmunds lost weight recently? What is her appetite like? Find out what she likes and dislikes with food and fluid so that these can be encouraged.
   • **Elimination** Limited exercise, loss of appetite and pyrexia may lead to constipation. Discover if this is a problem for Mrs Edmunds and if she has a remedy of her own.
   • **Rest and sleep** Find out if Mrs Edmunds has problems in this area due to pain and/or discomfort. Does she have any methods of overcoming sleeplessness?

2 The nurse should pay particular attention to the following:
   • **Comfort**
     1 A bedcradle will keep bedclothes off painful joints.
     2 Bedclothes should be lightweight.
     3 Mrs Edmunds should be given a daily wash and a hand and face wash whenever she feels hot and uncomfortable.
   • **Relief of pain**
     1 Analgesia should be given as prescribed.
     2 Careful positioning and handling are necessary.

- **Relief of stress**
  1 The patient must be given time to express anxieties and feelings.
    2 Support and encouragement should be offered.

3

Feature	Osteoarthritis	Rheumatoid arthritis
Type of condition	Degenerative	Inflammatory
Joints involved	Usually weight-bearing joints	Usually smaller joints
Extent of features	Clinical features confined to joint(s) affected	Systemic features as well as joint manifestations
Pathology	Degeneration of articular cartilage ↓ Development of bone spurs ↓ Roughened joints	Thickening of synovial membrane ↓ Growth of granulation tissue ↓ Erosion of articular cartilage
	→ Pain ←	
	Limited movement	
	Stiffness and deformity	

Draw up a table as shown above and see how much your junior colleague can fill in by herself before explaining the main differences and completing the chart.

4 - Reassure Mr Edmunds that this type of arthritis is not caused by cold or damp.
   - Explain that the exact cause is not yet known but that theories as to the cause include:
     1 a viral agent
     2 inherited factors
     3 disordered immunity
     4 psychological stress (may be a factor in worsening the condition)

Try to discover if Mr Edmunds thinks this is possible and what he feels is the cause of the stress.

- It is important that you can offer support at this stage if Mr Edmunds is still blaming himself for his wife's condition.
5
- The bed should have a firm mattress to support Mrs Edmunds' body.
- She should have one soft pillow so that her neck is in alignment with the rest of her body.
- Resting splints (plastic or plaster of Paris back-slabs) will rest the joints in the greatest possible extension without causing pain. (Joints limited in function tend to flex.)
- A bedcradle will take the weight of the bedclothes off the joints, thus preventing foot drop.
- Mrs Edmunds' limbs should be positioned carefully in the optimum position.
- Daily passive exercises should be carried out, putting all joints through a full range of movements.

6

Drug	Side-effects	Care
Indomethacin	Severe indigestion, gastrointestinal upsets, peptic ulcer Mental confusion, light-headedness, skin rash	• Take with or after meals and take milk at bedtime. • Ask Mrs Edmunds to report these occurrences.
Dihydro-codeine	Constipation, tolerance and dependence sedation.	• Provide 2–3 litres of fluid daily. • Provide a high fibre diet • Vary analgesia if these side-effects become troublesome.
Ferrous sulphate	Gastrointestinal upsets, constipation	• Provide 2–3 litres of fluid daily. • Provide a high fibre diet. • Vary analgesia if these side-effects become troublesome.

7   Appropriate exercise can preserve and sometimes increase joint mobility by preventing ankylosis, maintaining muscle tone and improving strength and mobility.

Only gentle exercise should be encouraged and the nurse should be careful not to overtire Mrs Edmunds. When joints are exercised too vigorously, dislocation may occur.

All joints should be put through their full range of movement at least once daily depending on the severity of each joint.

Occupational therapy can also help to restore joint mobility in the hands. Needlework, leatherwork, weaving or printing are particularly useful.

Hydrotherapy is useful for mobility of larger joints. Patients find they can move their limbs easily and painlessly under water, which also helps morale.

8   **Help**
  * A home help can do heavy shopping and housework.
  * A community nurse may be necessary if help with bathing is needed.
  * Aids for daily living can be supplied by the occupational therapy department.
  * Alterations can be made to the home to allow Mrs Edmunds to be as active and as independent as possible.

Advice
  * Take medication as prescribed. [You should warn of side-effects and what to do about these (see ans. 7) and provide easy-to-open bottles.]
  * Continue to exercise all joints daily. Expect some discomfort but do not persevere to the point of pain and fatigue.
  * Avoid long periods of immobility to prevent stiffness (e.g. stop on long drives to stretch legs).
  * Avoid sitting in low, deep armchairs. Upright chairs prevent excessive bending at the hip and support the back.

You should explain that rheumatoid arthritis has spontaneous remissions and that psychological stress can exacerbate the condition.

Further Reading

General nursing

Brunner, L. & Suddarth, D. (1982) *The Lippincott Manual of Medical–Surgical Nursing*. Vol. 1–3. London: Harper & Row.

Clark, J. E., Sage, C. A. & Attree, M. J. (1985) *Revise Essential Nursing Care*, Letts Study Aids. London: Charles Letts & Co.

Faulkner, A. (1985) *Nursing—A Creative Approach*. London: Baillière Tindall.

Hunt, P. & Sendell, B. (1984) *Nursing the Adult with a Specific Physiological Disturbance*. London: The Macmillan Press.

Long, B. C. & Phipps, W. J. (1985) *Essentials of Medical–Surgical Nursing*. St Louis: C.V. Mosby.

Parkin, D. (1985) *Revise Nursing RGN*, Letts Study Aids. London: Charles Letts & Co.

Roper, N., Logan, W. & Tierney, A. (1985) *The Elements of Nursing*. Edinburgh: Churchill Livingstone.

The Royal Marsden Hospital (1984) In Pritchard, A. & Walker, V. A. (eds.) *Manual of Clinical Nursing Policies and Procedures*. London: Harper & Row.

Specific to topics included in this book

Carey, K. (Ed.) (1984) *Hypertension*. Nursing Now Series. Pennsylvania: Springhouse Corporation.

Clarke, D. (1982) *Mentally Handicapped People*. London: Baillière Tindall.

Hamilton, H. (Ed.) (1985) *Gastrointestinal Disorders*, Nurses Clinical Library. Pennsylvania: Springhouse Corporation.

Mourad, L. (1980) *Nursing Care of Adults with Orthopaedic Conditions*. New York: John Wiley & Sons.

Urosevich, P. (Ed.) (1978) *Managing Diabetes Properly*. Nursing Skillbook. Pennsylvania: Intermed Communications.

Wilson, V. (1983) *Cardiac Nursing*. Oxford: Blackwell Scientific Publications.